STAY YOUNGER | LIVE LONGER

Healing Superfoods for Anti-Aging

KAREN ANSEL, MS, RDN, CDN

HEARST
books

HEARSTBOOKS

An Imprint of Sterling Publishing Co., Inc.
1166 Avenue of the Americas
New York, NY 10036

ISBN 978-1-61837-228-4

Distributed in Canada by Sterling Publishing Co., Inc.
c/o Canadian Manda Group, 664 Annette Street
Toronto, Ontario, Canada M6S 2C8
Distributed in the United Kingdom by GMC Distribution Services
Castle Place, 166 High Street, Lewes, East Sussex, England BN7 1XU
Distributed in Australia by NewSouth Books
45 Beach Street, Coogee, NSW 2034, Australia

For information about custom editions, special sales, and premium
and corporate purchases, please contact Sterling Special Sales at
800-805-5489 or specialsales@sterlingpublishing.com.

Manufactured in China

2 4 6 8 10 9 7 5 3 1

www.sterlingpublishing.com

Photo credits: © James Baigrie: O (bottom right); © Monica Buck: O (top); © Steve Giralt: P;
© Lisa Hubbard: J; iStock: © Almaje: B (bottom left); © Annalleysh: C; © doris2712: L;
© Julia_Sudnitskaya: B (bottom right); © Lilechka75: O (bottom left); © Lauri Patterson: B (top);
© Kate Mathis: F, G (left), K (top), M; © Marcus Nilsson: A; Courtesy Oldways and the Whole Grains
Council, wholegrainscouncil.org: 33; © Con Poulos: D, N; © Kate Sears: I, K (bottom left); StockFood:
© People Pictures: K (bottom right); © Kat Teusch: E; © Jonny Valiant: G (right); © Anna Williams: H

Book design by Anna Christian

CONTENTS

PART ONE

STOP THE CLOCK FROM THE INSIDE OUT

CHAPTER 1

Your User's Guide

Imagine a healthier you—with glowing skin, stronger hair and nails, more energy, and lower risk of disease. It's possible. And the solution is as close as your kitchen!

If you've ever tried to lose weight in a hurry, just to gain it all back, you know that crash diets, juice fasts, and other quick-fix weight loss methods don't work. Initially, the pounds might fall off, but up to two-thirds of dieters regain the lost weight within 4 or 5 years. The reason? Restrictive fad diets are hard to stick with for the long haul, so eventually people revert to their old eating habits—and the pounds creep back on. So, you'll be happy to learn that this book is *not* a diet plan. Rather, it's an easy-to-use guide to choosing the 101 top age-erasing foods, or Power Foods, which are brimming with Super Nutrients that will help you look and feel better than you have in years.

Drawing on decades of science and recipe testing, this book offers up nearly one hundred simple, delicious meal, snack, and dessert how-tos. It doesn't require eating mountains of broccoli or kale, or shopping for strange ingredients at a health food store either. You can buy every single item in the pages that follow in your supermarket. Most of the recipes take less than 35 minutes to prepare (and some are as quick as 15 minutes!).

There are no extremes. The focus is on balance. What really matters is the bigger picture: your overall health.

THE *HEALING SUPERFOODS FOR ANTI-AGING* PROMISE

Make the foods in this book the foundation of your diet, and you can expect:

◆ A healthier heart, including lower blood pressure and lower levels of cholesterol and triglycerides, a kind of fat found in your blood.

◆ Reduced risk of type 2 diabetes, thanks to more balanced blood sugar and insulin levels.
◆ Protection against cancer.
◆ A sharper memory, a better mood, and a sounder night's sleep.
◆ Stronger bones and muscles.
◆ Younger-looking skin, including fewer fine lines.
◆ Thicker, healthier hair and nails, plus a brighter smile.

Along the way, you'll become an expert in the Super Nutrients and the Power Foods you need to defy time. In fact, you may see some Super Nutrients more than once, though for different reasons. That's because many of them do double (or even triple!) duty. Consider protein. It keeps your muscles strong, builds bones, *and* helps your skin stay supple. You'll learn why you need it for each of these functions—and the smartest Power Foods to do the job.

ABOUT THE AUTHOR

Where did this ultimate collection of rejuvenating ingredients come from? Nutritionist and *Woman's Day* contributing editor Karen Ansel, MS, RDN, CDN, selected the Power Foods and their corresponding recipes, then created the meal plans in each chapter. The food is real, delicious, filling, and whole—not a bunch of overly processed snacks or pricey "diet" food. You should never feel deprived by incorporating them into your day-to-day meals.

In a world where you're being told to cut carbs, sugar, fat, salt, and gluten (often, all at the same time!), it can be difficult to know *how* to eat right. In the *Nutritionist's note* in each chapter, Karen will help you navigate food and health trends as she weighs in on the diet concerns she hears from women just like you.

HOW THIS BOOK WORKS

Each chapter focuses on key Super Nutrients to keep you younger and healthier, such as flavonoids to fight cancer or magnesium for better blood sugar. You'll also learn about certain Power Foods that contain these nutrients, like grapefruit for flavonoids, and brown rice for magnesium. Then, sprinkled throughout each chapter, you'll find these nuggets of advice:

➤ QUICK IDEAS No-fuss mini-recipes that show you ways to use each Power Food

➤ SMART TIPS Easy food-prep tricks and storage tips to help you work more Super Nutrients onto your plate

➤ FACTS The latest studies and stats on eating to turn back the clock

➤ GOOD TO KNOW! Helpful information about how each Power Food and Super Nutrient halts the aging process

➤ DID YOU KNOW? Surprising ways Power Foods and Super Nutrients boost longevity

➤ BONUS! The Power Foods in this book are filled with a multitude of health-promoting nutrients and benefits. Read all about them here.

In addition, the following chapter components provide even more pointers to putting anti-aging eating into action:

➤ THE TRUTH ABOUT . . . A closer look at food crazes, from coconut oil to cleanses

➤ EAT SMART Genius advice on topics such as how to spot hidden sugars in food and ways to avoid foods that spoil your smile

➤ DOWNSIZE IT! Tricks on cutting down on salt, eating less red meat, and more

➤ LIQUID ASSETS Information about your favorite drinks—which ones are best for you, and which ones are best in moderation

➤ ALL ABOARD! Wish your family ate more healthfully? Here's how to win over even the pickiest eaters.

If you've ever wondered if a vegetarian diet can prevent cancer, or if eggs can be part of a heart-healthy diet, you'll find the answers here.

➤ HABIT REHAB Learn simple strategies to nip unwanted behaviors in the bud.

➤ RECIPES Tasty breakfast, lunch, dinner, dessert, and snack recipes using the Power Foods in each chapter—locate the recipes themselves in chapter 9.

Last, the *Food label sleuth* explanations will show you how to navigate the Nutrition Facts panel on popular packaged foods. Even

HOW CAN I EASILY TELL WHAT A MEASUREMENT IS?

Here's how some common serving sizes look:

MEASURE	IS THE SIZE OF A . . .
1 teaspoon	Water bottle cap
1 tablespoon	Poker chip
2 tablespoons	Table tennis ball
1/4 cup	Large egg
1/2 cup	Regular cupcake liner
1 cup	Baseball

though this label is filled with valuable information, it's not always that easy to decipher. Use these simple steps to translate the panels' facts and figures:

Maintaining a healthy body weight is one of the very best things you can do to look and feel your youngest. The serving size at the top of the Nutrition Facts panel can help.

Also, be sure to read the *servings per container* stat, as the more servings you eat, the more calories you consume (specifically, the calories figure is the number of calories in a single serving).

The *Daily Value* is an estimate of how much of a nutrient—from fiber to fat—the average person needs each day. (This book, however, focuses on your Recommended Dietary Allowance, which is broken down by age and gender and gives a much more relevant amount of a nutrient you require.) When it comes to vitamins and minerals on the Nutrition Facts panel, like *vitamin D, calcium, iron,* or *potassium,* their Daily Values are given as a percentage. Consider 5 percent a low amount; 20 percent or more is high.

The *ingredient list* can be your best friend when it comes to sorting out what's *really* inside your favorite foods. It doesn't reveal exactly how much of each ingredient is in a product, but it does list each ingredient from greatest to least by weight

PUTTING IT ALL TOGETHER

To help you eat as many of the 101 Power Foods as possible, you'll find a one-week meal plan at the end of every chapter. Depending on your goals you can customize this plan to lose weight or keep your weight steady. If you have a few pounds to spare, you'll likely drop a couple of pounds a month (or more, if you're active!). This kind of slow, steady weight loss means you'll never have to worry about yo-yo dieting or regaining those hard-earned lost pounds.

Each day provides a base of 1,500 calories. You'll start with a nourishing 300-calorie breakfast, refuel with 400 calories for lunch, and end the day with a satisfying 500-calorie dinner. To stay full between meals, you can indulge in two 150-calorie snacks. If you're very active or weight loss isn't your goal, feel free to eat three snacks. And, if you're a man who's also trying to shed a few pounds—or there's one in your life—it's also okay to add in one additional snack a day, as men tend to be bigger and burn more calories. Men who are particularly active can indulge in two snacks that are double in size, rather than three regular-size snacks.

You won't find any of the restrictive diet advice that makes many popular weight loss plans so difficult to follow—just delicious, well-balanced eating advice. And the meal plans throughout the book are flexible, too. Each meal is roughly equal in calories, so you can mix, match, or repeat them in any order you like. If you're following a special diet, such as one that's gluten-free, low-carb, or vegetarian, chapter 9 has a meal plan designed especially for you. There, you'll also find a master meal plan that's chock full of the age-delaying Power Foods and Super Nutrients in this book.

Now that you've learned how to approach *Superfoods for Anti-Aging,* turn the page and start eating for a more youthful, healthier you!

READY, SET, SUCCESS!

As you read this book, you'll be inspired to make some powerful changes. But eating better doesn't happen overnight. These nine steps can help you use the advice in this book to develop new habits that will last a lifetime.

1 **Pick your top three goals.** When you're motivated to improve your health, it's normal to want to shake everything up at once. Yet you'll have more success if you prioritize. Researchers at Cornell University found that people who consistently made just three diet changes, such as portioning food onto plates instead of eating out of the package, using smaller plates, or drinking water with meals, had the most health-boosting benefits.

2 **Write it down.** There's a reason nutritionists are big fans of food journals: they exponentially increase your awareness of exactly what you're eating. Food logs are so effective, they've been shown to double the odds of weight-loss success, if that's your goal.

3 **Shake up your routine.** If you nibble on cookies every night while watching TV, maybe it's the TV, not the cookies, that's the problem. Why? Your brain has learned to expect a sweet snack when you flip on your favorite show. Switch to a different activity in another room, like reading a book in the family room instead, and kicking your cookie habit will become a whole lot easier.

4 **Hang out with the right pals.** Whether you want to eat more fruits and vegetables, drink less soda, or simply move more, research reveals that people tend to eat and exercise like their friends. Spend more time with people who inspire you, and you'll begin to internalize their healthy habits.

5 **Make it automatic.** It's hard to eat right when you barely have time to eat at all. For hectic days or nights, stock your freezer with healthy frozen meals that you can grab in a pinch (for options, turn to page 19 in chapter 2). One study found people who chose a single-serve frozen lunch over a restaurant lunch trimmed a hefty 374 calories per day.

6 **Distract yourself.** Your cravings may seem insatiable, but the truth is they come and go. The best way to conquer yours is to distract yourself with a new activity, such as walking the dog, painting your nails, or helping the kids with homework.

7 **Hide it.** The more effort it takes to eat a food, the less likely you are to want it. Ideally, it would be great if you could purge your kitchen of all less-than-healthy snacks and sweets, but that might not be practical for the rest of your family. If you need to keep a few tempting nibbles in the house, tuck them away where you're least likely to see them.

8 **Give it time.** You may have heard that it takes 21 days to change a habit. Not so, say experts at London's Cancer Research UK Health Behaviour Research Centre. They found that the amount of time to build better behaviors varied from as little as 18 days for some people to as long as 254 days for others.

9 **Practice, practice, practice.** When it comes to learning anything new, repetition is key. The best way to retrain your brain to develop any longevity-boosting behavior? Practice it every single day.

CHAPTER 2

Have a Healthier Heart

Heart disease takes the lives of more women than all forms of cancer combined. The sooner you adopt a heart-friendly diet, the lower your risk—and the bigger the benefits.

HOW HEART DISEASE DEVELOPS

When it comes to living a long, active life, few things are as important as having a strong, healthy heart. Even if you feel perfectly fine now, avoiding heart disease should be high on your list of priorities, because the disease develops slowly over a lifetime. A staggering 90 percent of American women have at least one risk factor. Yet they don't always know it, as symptoms in women differ from those in men and are easily confused with other illnesses.

One of the greatest contributors to heart troubles is high cholesterol. While you need some cholesterol for optimal health (see "Helpful vs. Harmful Cholesterol" on page 11), too much can combine with fats and proteins in your bloodstream to form a substance known as plaque, which can coat your arteries and cause them to narrow. Over time, this makes it harder for blood to flow to your heart. And if the plaque breaks apart, it can cause a blood clot to form, potentially blocking an artery completely and leading to a heart attack.

HELPFUL VS. HARMFUL CHOLESTEROL

Cholesterol is a waxy material that's in every cell of your body. And even though cholesterol gets a lot of bad press, your body *requires* it to make vitamin D, certain hormones, and other substances that help you digest food. But some types of blood cholesterol are better for you than others. The beneficial kind, known as HDL, or high-density lipoprotein, is like your body's cholesterol disposal system. HDL scours your bloodstream for unneeded cholesterol and ferries it back to your liver, where

it's broken down for other jobs or eliminated entirely. The other form of cholesterol, LDL, or low-density lipoprotein, is more prone to accumulate in your arteries and cause plaque to build up. How to remember which is which? Shorten LDL to L, as in, the type of cholesterol you want to *lower*, and think of HDL as H, the type you want to have *higher*.

THE GOOD NEWS

Eating foods with age-defying nutrients can keep your heart in peak condition by controlling cholesterol levels, blood pressure, and fats in your blood known as triglycerides. In addition to focusing on the right foods, it's important to eat them in the proper amounts to maintain a healthy body weight. Excess pounds put a strain on your heart and can lead to type 2 diabetes, which dramatically increases your odds of developing heart troubles. Staying active helps manage body weight, lower blood pressure, and reduce harmful LDL cholesterol, while boosting good HDL cholesterol. But that doesn't mean you have to sweat it out at for hours at the gym! According to the Centers for Disease Control, as little as three brisk 10-minute walks 5 days a week can benefit your heart.

SUPER NUTRIENTS AND POWER FOODS
MONOUNSATURATED FATS

What They Are: Monounsaturated fats (or MUFAs, as health experts like to call them) are a kind of fat that's especially good for your heart. Cooking oils that are rich in these fats, like canola and olive oil, are fluid at room

---

TOP 10 RISK FACTORS
for heart disease

- ◆ An unhealthy diet
- ◆ High blood pressure
- ◆ Diabetes and prediabetes
- ◆ Being overweight
- ◆ Smoking
- ◆ A sedentary lifestyle
- ◆ Being older than 55
- ◆ A family history of heart disease
- ◆ Elevated LDL cholesterol
- ◆ Heavy drinking

CHOLESTEROL BY THE NUMBERS

Nearly half of all American women have either borderline high risk or full-blown high risk cholesterol. And it's more likely to creep up as you age. In addition to watching your cholesterol levels, you'll want to keep an eye on triglycerides. Too many of these can raise your odds of a heart attack as well. Here's how to put your numbers into perspective:

	IDEAL	BORDERLINE HIGH RISK	HIGH RISK
Total cholesterol	< 200 mg/dL	200-239 mg/dL	> 240 mg/dL
LDL cholesterol	<100 mg/dL*	130-159 mg/dL	> 160 mg/dL
HDL cholesterol	> 60mg/dL	40-59 mg/dL**	< 40 mg/dL
Triglycerides	< 150 mg/dL	150-199 mg/dL	> 200 mg/dL

*Near ideal LDL cholesterol is 100-129 mg/dL (milligrams per deciliter).

**Note: This range isn't considered to be a risk, it's just that a level above 60mg/dL can actually help *protect* against heart disease.

temperature—a visual tipoff that they're heart-friendly. On the flip side, fats that are solid at room temperature, like butter, cheese, and coconut oil, are rich in saturated fats, a kind of fat that's considered to be problematic for heart health because it makes your body produce extra LDL cholesterol.

How They Improve Heart Health: The latest research proves that the type of fat on your plate is far more important than the amount. In fact, the American Heart Association says that it's okay to get up to 25–35 percent of your calories from fat—as long as you limit saturated fat, from foods like red meat, full-fat cheese, and whole milk, in favor of healthier monounsaturated and polyunsaturated fats. Like monounsaturated fats, polyunsaturated fats are found mainly in plant foods, especially soybeans, nuts, and sunflower, pumpkin, and sesame seeds. However, monounsaturated fats are the most

TRANS FAT ALERT

Thanks to a labeling loophole, foods can claim they're trans-fat-free even if they contain up to 0.5 gram of these unhealthy fats. That might not sound like much, but if you eat more than one serving those numbers quickly multiply. To be sure, comb the ingredient list for the term "partially hydrogenated fat," the technical name for trans fats.

advantageous, as they protect good HDL, while polyunsaturated fats can lower it.

FACT: Cheese is the top source of saturated fat in the American diet.

GOOD TO KNOW! According to the Mayo Clinic, every six pounds you drop can raise your HDL by 1 milligram per deciliter.

Where to Find Them:
AVOCADOS

Avocados may be rich in fat, but 66 percent of that fat is the beneficial monounsaturated variety. One note: A single avocado contains about 320 calories, so keep serving sizes to about a quarter of an avocado.

➤ QUICK IDEA For a healthy snack, mash a quarter of an avocado and spread it on a small warmed corn tortilla.

➤ BONUS! Avocados provide fiber, another nutrient that's key for a healthy heart. One quarter of an avocado gives you 3.5 grams of fiber.

➤ SMART TIP You can help an avocado ripen faster by storing it in a paper bag with an apple or a banana.

———

RECIPES
◆ Avocado Chicken, page 159

FOOD LABEL SLEUTH
Fat and cholesterol

Total fat is the amount of fat in grams per serving. You'll also see this listed as a percentage of the Daily Value from fat. As you may remember from chapter 1, the Daily Value estimates the amount of a nutrient that the average person should consume for good health. The trouble is that this figure is based on a 2,000-calorie diet. Considering that most women don't need this many calories, the Daily Value for fat may overstate how much you actually need. Instead, it may be more helpful to aim for a range of fat of about 40 (if you're petite) to 70 grams a day (if you're tall), from mainly mono- and polyunsaturated sources.

More important than total fat are the figures for saturated and trans fats. Trans fats are made by adding hydrogen to vegetable oil to make it more solid and extend its shelf life. The concern is that those newfangled fats elevate unhealthy LDL cholesterol and lower helpful HDL cholesterol. Since no amount of trans fat is considered safe, try your best to avoid it completely (see "Trans Fat Alert" on page 12). As for saturated fat? You don't need to eliminate it from your plate entirely, but for optimal heart health you should limit it to no more than 10 percent of your total calories, or about 17-20 grams a day.

For the reasons already discussed, it's not necessary to obsess about cholesterol. If you have existing heart troubles, speak with your doctor about how much is right for you.

If you've suddenly noticed that coconut oil is being praised as the latest miracle food, it's not your imagination. For years, the saturated fat–filled oil topped the diet don't list for heart health. Suddenly, it seems like books and websites everywhere are promoting it to fight heart disease and cancer and even boost metabolism.

Why the about-face? Since most plant oils are made of predominantly mono- and polyunsaturated fats, coconut oil (along with palm oil) is unique in that it's mostly saturated fat. Health experts originally assumed that because coconut oil's fat was almost entirely saturated, it spelled bad news for our hearts. They now know that coconut oil is made of a mix of several different kinds of saturated fats. While many of these are unfriendly to your heart, slightly more than half of them have little effect on your LDL cholesterol.

➤ **BOTTOM LINE:** Until there's more research, stick with safer picks like olive and canola oils for frying or sautéeing. For baking, coconut oil is probably no better or worse for you than butter, but since both of these are high in saturated fat, it's safest to use them sparingly.

+ Avocado Swiss Breakfast Sandwich, page 137
+ Black Bean Burger Salad, page 149
+ Mexican Burrito Bowl, page 188

OLIVE OIL

Olive oil is exceptionally rich in monounsaturated fat. But that's only one of the reasons it's so good for your cardiovascular health. Olive oil is also packed with polyphenols, plant substances that may raise HDL cholesterol and help manage LDL cholesterol. How so? LDL cholesterol is susceptible to attacks by damaging compounds called free radicals. This process, known as oxidation, can change LDL cholesterol's composition, making it even more harmful to your blood vessels. By eating more olive oil, you'll load up on polyphenols that prevent oxidation.

➤ **GOOD TO KNOW!** Cocoa and green tea also contain plenty of polyphenols.

➤ **SMART TIP** Choose extra virgin olive oil for salads and uncooked dishes. It's less processed than refined olive oil, so it retains more ticker-friendly polyphenols than regular or virgin varieties. High temperatures destroy delicate polyphenols, though, so regular olive oil is fine for sautéeing or frying.

OMEGA-3 FATS

What They Are: Omega-3 fats are special kinds of polyunsaturated fat found in fatty fish and a small number of plant foods. In addition to improving your cardiovascular health, they help keep your cells healthy, especially cells in your brain and eyes, and they may guard against dementia and depression.

How They Improve Heart Health: These favorable fats help regulate your heart rhythms, protecting against irregular heartbeats, which can be fatal. They also prevent plaque buildup by lowering triglycerides.

There are two kinds of omega-3s. The first kind is the long-chain omega-3s, DHA (docosapentaenoic acid) and EPA (eicosapentaenoic acid). You can get these from eating fish. And there's another kind of shorter-chain omega-3: ALA (alpha linolenic acid). If you're not a big fan of fish, you can get the ALA variety from plant foods such as flaxseed, chia seed, walnuts, and canola oil. The slight drawback? Your body has to turn ALA into longer-chain omega-3s before it can use it, and only about 15 percent is converted into EPA and DHA. Since health experts recommend you consume 1,100 milligrams of ALA each day, put plant Power Foods into the regular rotation.

➤ FACT Nearly a third of Americans have borderline high triglycerides, making triglyceride-lowering omega-3s especially important.

➤ GOOD TO KNOW! Just one or two fish meals a week can slash your risk of sudden cardiac death from irregular heartbeats in half.

Where to Find Them:
CANOLA OIL
Like olive oil, canola oil is a top source of monounsaturated fat—1 tablespoon delivers more ALA than you need in an entire day. It's also one of the few foods that provide meaningful amounts of plant omega-3s. That's key, since most people don't get enough of these beneficial fats. (Instead, most of the fats Americans eat come from another type of less-healthy polyunsaturated fat known as omega-6 fats, which are frequently used in packaged and processed foods.) Canola's neutral flavor works well in just about any dish. Swap it in for vegetable oil when cooking.

➤ DID YOU KNOW? Canola oil has less saturated fat than other cooking oils.

THREE TRICKS TO WORK MORE PLANT FATS ONTO YOUR PLATE

➤ FACT: As little as two-and-a-half daily servings of vegetables have been shown to trim heart disease risk by an impressive 23 percent. No, you don't have to go full-blown vegetarian or vegan. But swapping more plant-based fats into your lineup will help your heart.

Try these easy ideas:

1 **At breakfast, skip the margarine or butter,** and spread one-quarter of a mashed avocado onto whole-wheat toast.

2 **Shake up your peanut butter habit,** and experiment with other nut and seed spreads. Then, instead of having a turkey or ham sandwich for lunch, make a sunflower-, hazelnut-, or almond-butter-and-banana one.

3 **Choose a better bar.** Energy bars can be a smart snack to stash in your bag, desk drawer, or car for hunger emergencies. For the best picks, look for brands that list nuts or fruit as the first ingredient and contain no more than 200 calories, 3 grams of saturated fat, and 12-15 grams of sugar.

➤ **BONUS!** One tablespoon of canola oil gives you 16 percent of your daily dose of vitamin E, another heart-supporting nutrient.

CHIA SEEDS

These little seeds are big on short-chain ALA omega-3s. A whopping 58 percent of their fat comes from ALA. Just 1 tablespoon of chia seeds gives you more than 2,000 milligrams (roughly twice your daily dose).

➤ **QUICK IDEA** For an instant omega-3 boost, sprinkle some chia seeds into your salad, oatmeal, cereal, or yogurt.

➤ **SMART TIP** When you put chia seeds into liquid, they swell up and turn into small jelly-like balls. Swirl 1 tablespoon of chia seeds into iced tea or juice to transform a drink into a satisfying snack.

➤ **BONUS!** Chia seeds are rich in slowly digested protein and fiber, nutrients that work together to keep you full for hours. One ounce (slightly more than 2 tablespoons) gives you 10 grams of fiber and 5 grams of protein.

RECIPES
- Chia Pudding, page 224
- Sunrise Smoothie, page 144

FOOD LABEL SLEUTH
Sodium

Along with saturated and trans fat, sodium is another essential heart-health number. What's a safe amount? For most people, up to 2,300 milligrams a day. However, 1,500 milligrams may be more appropriate if you have heart issues or high blood pressure.

In case you're wondering how that translates to the food you eat, here's what milligrams look like in teaspoons of salt:

600 milligrams = 1/4 teaspoon of salt
1,200 milligrams = 1/2 teaspoon of salt
2,400 milligrams = 1 teaspoon of salt

YOU ASKED
Can eggs be part of a heart-healthy diet?

Yes! For a long time, health experts thought that too much cholesterol in food translated into high cholesterol in your blood. That's no longer the case. Since you need cholesterol to survive, your liver makes its own supply, churning out more than three times the amount of cholesterol you'd normally eat in a day. And your body is extremely clever. When you consume too much cholesterol, it balances things out by making less. Even though eggs pack a decent chunk of cholesterol (about 185 milligrams per large egg), health experts now agree that for healthy people one egg a day is completely fine. What's more, eggs are surprisingly low in saturated fat, at less than 2 grams per egg. If you don't have heart issues, go ahead and eat up. If you suffer from heart disease, high cholesterol, or diabetes, however, stick with a three-egg-a-week limit. Since cholesterol is found entirely in the yolk, you can eat as many egg whites as you like.

MAKE SENSE OF BLOOD PRESSURE NUMBERS

When your doctor takes your blood pressure, she's actually measuring two numbers, systolic and diastolic blood pressure. Systolic blood pressure, or the number on top, tells the amount of pressure in your arteries when your heart is beating. The bottom figure, known as diastolic blood pressure, reveals the pressure when your heart relaxes. The box below can help you determine whether your numbers fall into the normal, borderline high, or high range.

CATEGORY	SYSTOLIC		DIASTOLIC
Normal	< 120	and	< 80
Borderline High	120-139	or	80-89
High	>140	or	> 90

SALMON

How's this for an impressive stat? A 2013 Harvard study found that people with the highest levels of long-chain omega-3 fats in their blood were 27 percent less likely to die from heart disease, and they lived an average of 2 years longer than those with the lowest levels. And fatty fish is where it's at—salmon, in particular. The pink-fleshed fish has more omega-3 fats than almost any other catch in the sea: One 4-ounce serving of cooked wild Atlantic salmon dishes up nearly 2,100 milligrams of omega-3s. At your next barbeque, swap in salmon steaks for your sirloin, T-bone, or rib eye. Their meaty flavor will please even die-hard carnivores.

➤ SMART TIP Farmed salmon can contain antibiotics, which may lead to antibiotic resistance. Stick with wild salmon whenever possible.

➤ GOOD TO KNOW! Trout, sardines, and herring are also packed with omega-3s.

➤ QUICK IDEA No time to cook? Fold drained canned salmon into salads or pasta. One 4-ounce serving contains up to 1,200 milligrams of these healthy fats.

➤ DID YOU KNOW? While baked, grilled, or broiled fish can fend off heart disease, eating just one serving of fried fish a week can up your risk of heart failure by 48 percent.

➤ BONUS! Salmon is a top source of bone-strengthening vitamin D. One 4-ounce fillet supplies nearly your entire day's worth.

➤ RECIPES

◆ Lemon Pasta with Salmon and Asparagus, page 180
◆ Salmon Pesto Sandwich, page 155
◆ Salmon Cakes, page 194

POTASSIUM

What It Is: Potassium is a mineral that helps regulate your body's fluid balance so that you don't become dehydrated. It also helps muscles contract, controls your heartbeat, and is involved in transmitting nerve signals. Without enough, you may develop muscle cramps and feel weak and nauseated.

Sodium

It's easy to blame the saltshaker for a sodium-heavy diet. Yet three-quarters of the sodium most people eat actually comes from restaurant and processed foods. At home, you can reduce sodium by choosing more fresh foods and fewer packaged ones. When cooking, ease up on added salt ("New Ways to Season to Taste" on page 135 in chapter 9 can show you how). For those times that you order in—or eat out—try these tips:

◆ **Say "no, thanks" to the breadbasket.** Bread may be the number one source of sodium on your plate. Not because each slice has so much, but because people tend to eat a *lot* of it. If you can't resist the smell of a fresh baked loaf, ask your server to take it away as soon as you sit down—or not to bring it at all.

◆ **Skip the soup.** Restaurant soups can be filled with sodium, so opt for a side salad instead. And be wary of canned varieties you pop open in a pinch. Stick with lower-sodium soups.

◆ **Cut down on cheese.** Whether it's on pizza, sandwiches, tacos, or burritos, cheese is oozing with sodium (not to mention saturated fat). Next time you dial out for pizza, ask for only half the amount of cheese and fill in the balance with vegetables. For sandwiches, tacos, or burritos, ask your server to leave it off. On pasta, skip the grated Parmesan as well—each heaping spoonful sneaks in close to 150 sodium milligrams. Chances are you'll never even know it's missing.

◆ **Go easy on the condiments.** Salad dressing, ketchup, barbecue sauce, and mustard all deliver sneaky sodium. Just two innocent packets of ketchup take up more than 10 percent of your total daily requirement. When possible, opt for oil and vinegar on your salad or use lemon juice as a seasoning. If you like things hot and spicy, ask for a shaker of crushed red pepper rather than salsa or hot sauce.

◆ **Think fresh.** When eating out, you may not be able to eliminate all of the sodium, but you can offset some of the damage. Instead of chips, ask for potassium-packed fruit as a side with your sandwich, or choose grilled vegetables as an appetizer.

◆ **Keep it simple.** The more ingredients in your dish, the more likely it is to contain sodium. Stick with single-ingredient menu items, like grilled fish or roast chicken. Also, don't be afraid to ask lots of questions about how your food will be prepared and request that added salt be left off.

➤ **DID YOU KNOW?** Seafood can be high in sodium. After all, most fish live in salt water, so they're literally swimming in it! But since seafood is among the healthiest foods for your heart, don't skimp on it. Focus your efforts instead on reducing sodium from other less-healthy foods. When buying canned fish such as tuna, choose reduced-sodium options.

How It Improves Heart Health: Potassium works to counteract the effects of sodium, a mineral found in salt. Left unchecked, sodium pulls water into your blood vessels, boosting blood pressure, which can damage blood vessel linings and cause blood clots to form. Considering that the average American eats more than 3,400 milligrams of sodium a day—nearly twice as much sodium as she needs—getting enough potassium is critical. Not only does potassium flush out excess sodium, it also keeps blood vessels relaxed and pliable, helping blood flow freely and easing the strain on your heart.

➤ **FACT** For optimal blood pressure and overall health, you should eat 4,700 daily milligrams of potassium. Most people don't reach half that amount.

➤ **DID YOU KNOW?** Your blood vessels become thicker and less flexible with age. As you get older, watching your sodium—and increasing potassium—becomes that much more critical.

Where to Find It:
LIMA BEANS

Haven't eaten lima beans since you were a kid (when Mom and Dad made you)? It's time to give them a second look. They're a top source of blood-pressure-lowering potassium, with 968 milligrams per cup. That may not sound like much, compared to your daily quota of 4,700 milligrams, but unlike many other nutrients, potassium is hard to get in big doses. That's one reason health experts suggest making produce half your plate—and loading up on potassium-rich plant foods like limas at every meal.

➤ **QUICK IDEA** Keep a bag of frozen limas in your freezer to add to low-sodium canned vegetable or tomato soup for an instant nutrition boost.

➤ **BONUS!** Lima beans are a surprising source of protein, with 12 grams per cup.

RECIPE
◆ Farmers Market Pasta, page 174

FOOD LABEL SLEUTH
Frozen meals

That little frozen lasagna may look like it's made for one person, but it could actually contain two or more servings. As mentioned in chapter 1, make the number of servings per container the first thing you look for.

◆ Pick meals with no more than 4 grams of saturated fat per serving.

◆ Your mission: find a meal that contains less than 600 milligrams of sodium.

◆ Anything with 3 or more grams of fiber per serving gets a thumbs-up.

◆ Any meal with 250 milligrams of potassium or more is a bonus.

The ingredients list is where you'll find out if your meal contains go-tos like whole grains, vegetables, fruit, and beans. But remember, when you see the words "partially hydrogenated," it means your meal is hiding cholesterol-raising trans fats.

NONFAT OR 1% MILK

If you want to lower your blood pressure in a hurry, a few daily servings of lowfat dairy could help do the trick. Researchers at the University of Texas at Austin put middle-aged volunteers with hypertension on a diet that included either four servings of nonfat dairy a day or four servings of applesauce, fruit cups, or fruit juice and *no* dairy for 1 month. After just 3 weeks, the dairy group's systolic blood pressure fell 6 percent. One reason may be milk's abundant potassium—the high-dairy diet provided 1,000 milligrams more of potassium a day than the processed fruit diet. And milk is a potassium powerhouse: one single cup contains 366 milligrams.

➤ **QUICK IDEA** Sneak more dairy into your diet by cooking whole grains like oatmeal in lowfat milk.

➤ **BONUS!** Dairy contains special milk proteins that help relax your arteries.

➤ **GOOD TO KNOW!** Raw milk and raw-milk cheese may sound healthy, but they can be swimming with dangerous bacteria, so proceed with caution.

ORANGES

Eating whole fruit is a sweet way to help your heart. In addition to providing potassium, one orange boasts 110 percent of your daily dose of vitamin C, needed to help your blood vessels contract and relax properly. It's also loaded with flavonoids, multitasking plant chemicals that keep your blood vessels healthy, ward off blood clots, and prevent LDL cholesterol oxidation (read more about flavonoids on page 51 in chapter 4). No wonder people who eat more citrus fruits

are less likely to experience a heart attack or stroke.

➤ **SMART TIP** Orange peel contains the blood pressure-lowering plant chemical hesperidin. Try grating orange zest into a beef and broccoli stir-fry, or swirling some into a vinaigrette.

RECIPES

- Beef Stir-Fry, page 160
- Orange and Apricot Quinoa, page 141
- Orange-Soy Tofu Stir-Fry, page 190
- Strawberry Smoothie, page 226

SOLUBLE FIBER

What It Is: When you think of fiber, chances are digestive health comes to mind. But better digestion is only one of the many ways fiber enhances your health. First, know that there are actually several different kinds of fiber, each with distinct benefits. The two main types are insoluble fiber and soluble fiber. Found in whole-wheat bread and bran, insoluble fiber (so called because it doesn't dissolve in water) pulls water into your digestive system, keeping you regular. Soluble fiber, from the likes of beans, peas, oats, and barley, dissolves in water and has been linked to major cardiovascular benefits.

How It Improves Heart Health: After you eat it, soluble fiber attaches to bile acids, cholesterol building blocks in your digestive system, and sweeps them out of your body. With fewer of these raw materials on hand to create cholesterol, there's less of a chance that cholesterol will clog your arteries. And that's not all. A fiber-filled diet is also shown to reduce levels of C-reactive protein, a marker of inflammation that can predict heart disease (your doctor can test for it). What exactly is inflammation? It's a sign that your body is trying to heal itself, like the way your finger becomes red and tender when you get a paper cut. A similar reaction can occur in your arteries when your body is trying to repair damage from plaque buildup.

➤ FACT A British Medical Journal analysis of 22 studies found that for every 7 grams of fiber a person ate a day, his or her odds of heart disease decreased by 9 percent.

➤ GOOD TO KNOW! Nutrition labels aren't required to tell you how much soluble fiber is in your favorite foods. Since roughly a third of fiber in food is soluble, eating 30 grams of total fiber a day should give you the 10 grams of soluble fiber you need for peak heart health.

➤ BONUS! Soluble fiber also helps regulate blood sugar by slowing down the rate sugar is absorbed into your bloodstream.

Where to Find It:
BARLEY
Roughly 30 percent of people have high LDL cholesterol—and barley can help lower it. Barley contains a special kind of soluble fiber known as beta glucan, which works like a vacuum, whooshing away the building blocks your body uses to make cholesterol. One way to get beta-glucan is to eat oatmeal every single day. But that can grow boring after a while. Instead, add some barley to your weekly menu. Research suggests it may be as effective at lowering cholesterol as oats.

NUTRITIONIST'S NOTE
On moderation

Often, when I talk to my clients about eating less of a certain food or nutrient, they assume that means they can't eat it at all. But advice to eat a low-salt diet doesn't mean you should try to adopt a no-salt diet. The same goes for saturated fat. With the exception of trans fats, there really aren't any foods, nutrients, or ingredients you need to nix completely. Even people with full-blown heart disease can consume up to 6 percent of their total calories from saturated fat, according to the American Heart Association. And while most people could benefit from less sodium, you actually need some of this mineral to survive.

➤ GOOD TO KNOW! Three grams of beta glucan a day is proven to help lower cholesterol. It's the amount in a heaping cup of cooked barley (or a big bowl of oatmeal).

➤ SMART TIP Cooked barley is a cinch to freeze. Simply whip up a big batch, divide it into single-serving plastic bags and freeze. That way, you'll always have some on hand to sprinkle into salads and soups.

RECIPES
◆ Barley-Stuffed Pepper, page 148
◆ Slow Cooker Butternut Squash Barley Risotto, page 197

EDAMAME

If there's one food that may help you live longer, it's beans. When researchers looked at the diets of five different cultures, they found that bean eaters were most likely to live the longest. While all beans are protective, edamame serves up special heart-health perks. In addition to being loaded with soluble fiber, these tasty soybeans are one of the only plant foods that supply complete protein like you'd get from meat, chicken, or fish. Even better, soy protein contains hardly any saturated fat and supplies a hefty dose of good-for-you mono- and polyunsaturated fats.

➤ QUICK IDEAS In addition to nibbling on edamame as a snack, use it to make hummus or toss it into rice dishes or stir-fries.

➤ GOOD TO KNOW! If you're trying to eat less meat, 1 cup of cooked edamame gives you 18 grams of protein.

➤ BONUS! Edamame are packed with potassium. One cup of shelled edamame provides 676 milligrams.

RECIPES

- Brown Rice Edamame Salad, page 151
- Orange-Soy Tofu Stir-Fry, page 190
- Soba Noodles with Shrimp, Snow Peas, Carrots, and Edamame, page 200
- Spicy Trail Mix, page 226

OTHER HEART-HEALTHY POWER FOODS

CRANBERRIES

How They Make Your Heart Healthier: They're rich in compounds that fight gum disease.

It may sound strange, but keeping your gums healthy is a smart line of defense for avoiding heart disease. Gum disease, or gingivitis, produces bacteria that travel from your mouth through your bloodstream to your arteries. There, the germs can cause damage that may favor the formation of blood clots. While nothing beats brushing and flossing daily, cranberries could give your gum health a boost, thanks to their ability to fight bacteria and prevent it from latching on to gum tissue.

➤ QUICK IDEA Mix fresh cranberries into oatmeal or use them to top pancakes or waffles.

➤ GOOD TO KNOW! Compared to fresh cranberries, which contain only 4 grams of sugar per cup, cranberry juice or dried cranberries can have added cavity-causing sugar. Check the ingredient list to be sure.

➤ BONUS! Cranberries provide heart-supporting vitamins C and E. And they're low in calories, at only 46 calories per cup.

RECIPE

- Tuna Fennel Wrap, page 156

PEARS

How They Make Your Heart Healthier: They're rich in flavanones.

Making sure your ticker stays in top condition isn't just about lowering cholesterol and triglycerides. Potent compounds in plants, known as phytonutrients, keep this muscle at its peak as well. Found in fruits, vegetables, beans, and whole grains, phytonutrients help blood vessels stay flexible and elastic, fight inflammation, and prevent blood clots that can cause blockages. One type that's especially good for your heart is flavanones—and pears are an excellent source.

➤ **GOOD TO KNOW!** You can also find flavanones in bran, apples, grapefruit, strawberries, and even red wine and chocolate.

➤ **FACT** A 2007 American Journal of Clinical Nutrition study found that women who ate pears or apples more than once a week were 15 percent less likely to die from heart disease than those who munched on these fruits less than once a week.

➤ **QUICK IDEA** Don't just save pears for snacking. Slice them into sandwiches and salads, too.

➤ **SMART TIP** Whip up a batch of pear sauce by substituting pears for apples in your favorite applesauce recipe. It's perfect on its own or stirred into yogurt, cottage cheese, or oatmeal.

➤ **BONUS!** Pears contain soluble fiber. One pear gives you a little more than 1 gram, or roughly 10 percent of your daily dose.

RECIPE
◆ Roasted Pears, page 219

PECANS
How They Make Your Heart Healthier: They're rich in polyphenols.

When it comes to nuts, walnuts and almonds seem to get all the love. But what about pecans? These rich, buttery nuts are a delicious way to work more helpful monounsaturated fats onto your plate. Beyond that, a 2011 Loma Linda University study found that pecans may protect against inflammation in your arteries. One reason could be pecans' polyphenols, plant substances that have been shown to lower blood pressure, improve cholesterol, and ease inflammation.

➤ **GOOD TO KNOW!** Edamame, green tea, parsley, and chocolate contain polyphenols as well.

HABIT REHAB
Salty Snacks

When you're watching your sodium, those milligrams can add up quickly. Whip up these painless swaps for popular packaged snacks:

INSTEAD OF: ¼ cup hummus and 10 pita chips
TRY: ¼ mashed avocado and 1 sliced red bell pepper
➤ **SODIUM SAVINGS:** 595 milligrams

INSTEAD OF: 15 small pretzels
TRY: 17 unsalted sweet potato chips
➤ **SODIUM SAVINGS:** 502 milligrams

INSTEAD OF: 2 cubes of Brie and 15 small whole-wheat crackers
TRY: 2 crisp breads with 2 tablespoons part-skim ricotta
➤ **SODIUM SAVINGS:** 99 milligrams

INSTEAD OF: 2 cups of lite microwave popcorn
TRY: 2 cups air-popped popcorn with a dash of curry powder or cinnamon
➤ **SODIUM SAVINGS:** 140 milligrams

➤ **QUICK IDEA** Toss toasted pecans into pasta with olive oil, roasted butternut squash, and wilted spinach.

➤ **SMART TIP** Pecans taste sweeter than most other nuts, so they're a healthy way to satisfy that craving for something decadent. The perfect portion is about 15 pecan halves with 155 calories and 16 grams of fat.

RECIPE

♦ Raisin Spice Breakfast Sundae, page 143

PISTACHIOS
How They Make Your Heart Healthier: They're rich in phytosterols.

Have you ever wondered how margarines and spreads that claim to lower your cholesterol work? They're enriched with plant sterols, substances that act like soluble fiber, blocking cholesterol absorption in your gut. You can also find phytosterols in nuts, especially pistachios.

➤ **GOOD TO KNOW!** Phytosterols are in many fruits, vegetables, seeds, beans, and grains, too.

➤ **FACT** Eating 2 grams of phytosterols a day can reduce your LDL by 6 to 15 percent without lowering desirable HDL cholesterol.

➤ **SMART TIP** Pistachios are a smart calorie bargain. You can eat a generous 49 of them for 160 calories. And shelling pistachios takes time—naturally slowing you down, so you feel full sooner.

RECIPE

♦ Beef Stir-Fry, page 160

SESAME SEEDS
How They Make Your Heart Healthier: They're also rich in phytosterols.

Don't love pistachios? Don't worry! Sesame seeds offer up more cholesterol-lowering phytosterols than any other nut or seed. With 1 gram of fiber in each tablespoon, they're an easy way to work some extra fiber onto your plate as well.

➤ **QUICK IDEAS** Use sesame seeds as a coating for baked sesame chicken, toss them into soba noodles with peanut sauce, or, for a double dose, sprinkle them on broccoli or snow peas sautéed in sesame oil.

➤ **DID YOU KNOW?** You can benefit from sesame's perks in tahini, a Middle Eastern spread made from sesame seeds. Try it instead of cream cheese on your whole-wheat bagel, toast, or English muffin for breakfast.

➤ **SMART TIP** To keep sesame seeds from turning rancid, store them tightly sealed in your pantry, for up to 3 months, or in your fridge for 6 months.

➤ **BONUS!** Sesame seeds are rich in calcium. Two tablespoons give you more of this bone-building mineral than half a glass of milk.

RECIPES

♦ Pepper-Crusted Tuna with Sesame Asparagus, page 192
♦ Sesame Salmon with Bok Choy, page 195

SPINACH
How It Makes Your Heart Healthier: It's rich in folate and antioxidants.

Spinach is a top source of folate, a B vitamin that prevents homocysteine, an amino acid linked to heart disease, from accumulating in your bloodstream (read about the good that amino acids do below and on page 89 in chapter 4). Just 1 cup of cooked spinach gives you two thirds of your day's worth of folate—around 40 calories. This leafy vegetable is also packed with antioxidants, substances that shield your LDL cholesterol from free radical attacks.

➤ QUICK IDEA Throw a few heaping cups of prewashed bagged spinach into a big salad. Not ready to give up your iceberg or romaine lettuce? Mix half lettuce and half spinach (you can do this with kale, too).

➤ BONUS! Spinach keeps your immune system strong, thanks to plenty of vitamins A and C.

———

RECIPES
+ Asian Chicken Tacos, page 147
+ Linguine with Tomatoes, Spinach, and Clams, page 183
+ Spinach-Feta Omelet, page 144

WATERMELON
How It Makes Your Heart Healthier: It's rich in citrulline.

Pliable, elastic arteries are important for cardiovascular health. And watermelon can help you achieve them. This juicy fruit is nature's number one source of citrulline, an amino acid that helps your body produce nitric oxide, a substance that keeps blood vessels supple and promotes blood flow. Considering that 60 percent of people have either prehypertension (the gray area right before you cross over into full-blown hypertension) or all-out high blood pressure, watermelon is a tasty way to keep your numbers in check.

➤ FACT When researchers at Florida State University fed prehypertensive volunteers citrulline-rich watermelon extract for 6 weeks, their arteries relaxed and their blood pressure improved as well.

➤ QUICK IDEA For a refreshing salad, toss chunks of watermelon with baby spinach and balsamic vinaigrette. Top with crushed pistachios.

➤ DID YOU KNOW? A cup of diced watermelon has only 46 calories.

➤ BONUS! Watermelon contains lycopene, a plant chemical that keeps your skin looking younger.

———

RECIPE
+ Watermelon Granita, page 221

One-week heart-healthy meal plan

	BREAKFAST	LUNCH	DINNER
DAY 1	Breakfast Burrito*	Couscous with Chickpeas*	1 medium baked potato with 2 tablespoons nonfat plain Greek yogurt or reduced-fat sour cream 1 cup broccoli sautéed in 1 teaspoon olive oil
DAY 2	1 slice whole wheat toast, topped with 2 tablespoons nut butter and 1/2 sliced pear	Brown Rice Edamame Salad*	Greek-Style Tilapia* 3/4 cup peas with 1 teaspoon olive oil Watermelon Granita*
DAY 3	Maple Almond Oatmeal	Black Bean Burger Salad* 1 cup cubed watermelon	Orange-Soy Tofu Stir Fry* 1/3 cup quinoa, prepared according to package directions
DAY 4	1 cup bran flakes with 1 tablespoon chopped pecans, 2 tablespoons unsweetened dried cranberries, and 1 cup 1% milk	Salmon Pesto Sandwich* Cantaloupe Cucumber Salad*	Mexican Burrito Bowl*
DAY 5	Raisin Spice Breakfast Sundae*	Barley Stuffed Pepper* 1 medium apple	Farmers Market Pasta*
DAY 6	Orange Apricot Quinoa*	Asian Chicken Tacos*	Pepper-Crusted Tuna with Sesame Asparagus* 1/4 cup brown rice, prepared according to package directions
DAY 7	Spinach-Feta Omelet* 1 medium orange	Spread 2 tablespoons nut butter and 1 tablespoon strawberry jam on an 8-inch whole-wheat pita. Top with 1/2 sliced banana. Fold into a wrap.	Chicken Vegetable Skewers* 1 serving Roasted Pears*

*Recipe included in chapter 9

Strawberry Smoothie*
45 pistachio nuts

½ cup grapes + 2 tablespoons pumpkin seeds
Unlimited broccoli and cauliflower florets dipped in 1 tablespoon ranch dressing

1 sliced bell pepper dipped in 1 tablespoon tahini
6 ounces nonfat plain Greek yogurt with ½ cup blueberries

Chocolate Chili Popcorn*
¼ cup part-skim ricotta mixed with 1 teaspoon fresh herbs (try parsley or tarragon) on 8 small whole-wheat crackers

15 pecan halves
12-ounce nonfat latte (6 ounces nonfat milk warmed in the microwave + 6 ounces hot brewed coffee) + 1 kiwi

1 apple + 1 tablespoon sunflower butter
¾ cup edamame

Spicy Trail Mix*
Chia Pudding*

CHECKLIST
For a healthier heart

❍ How to recall which form of cholesterol is harmful and which one is helpful? Think of LDL as L—the cholesterol number you want to *lower*—and HDL as H—the one you want to be *higher*.

❍ Whenever possible, replace saturated fats, which can raise undesirable LDL cholesterol, with monounsaturated and polyunsaturated fats.

❍ Choose olive and canola oils as your go-to cooking oils.

❍ Aim to eat at least two servings of fatty fish a week. Your best choices: salmon, trout, sardines, and herring.

❍ Downsize saturated fat by eating less red meat and full-fat dairy.

❍ For more potassium, eat at least one serving of fruits or vegetables with each meal and at most snacks. Beans and lowfat dairy can help you get more potassium, too.

❍ Work more soluble fiber into your meals with foods like beans, pears, apples, barley, and oatmeal.

❍ If your cholesterol is high, try to include more phytosterol-rich nuts and seeds (especially pistachios and sesame seeds) into meals and snacks.

❍ Sleuth out hidden sodium, saturated fat, and trans fats by reading food labels carefully.

❍ Don't forget to exercise, even if it's a few quick walks a day!

CHAPTER 3

Balance Blood Sugar for Good

In the past 30 years, new cases of diabetes have more than tripled. The right foods—in the right amounts— can help you beat the odds.

HOW DIABETES DEVELOPS

No doubt, you've heard of the hormone insulin. But what *exactly* does it have to do with diabetes? Insulin is a key that unlocks the door that lets sugar, or glucose, into your cells. Glucose is your body and brain's number one source of energy—the kind of energy that you need to live and breathe. When your body either doesn't produce enough insulin or has difficulty using the insulin it does generate, blood sugar builds up, and you can become diabetic.

There are actually several types of diabetes. The two most common kinds are type 1 and type 2. Type 1 usually strikes before adulthood and is an autoimmune disease in which your body mistakenly kills off special insulin-producing cells, known as beta cells, in the pancreas. Without enough beta cells, glucose starts to spiral out of control. Since type 1 diabetics can't generate insulin at all, they require insulin injections to stay alive.

People with type 2, however, tend to make insulin, but their bodies have trouble using it efficiently. While type 2 may seem to appear suddenly, it develops slowly, starting as a condition known as insulin resistance, which is caused by factors such as aging and weight gain, especially around your middle. Other than making your jeans too tight, this fat begins to manufacture compounds that can cause your body to be less responsive (or "sensitive," as experts say) to the insulin you produce. This results in a condition known as prediabetes, where blood sugar rises but not to the level of diabetes. Your pancreas tries

to help by making even more insulin—and eventually it wears out.

Usually, 15–30 percent of people with prediabetes will become diabetic within 5 years. Some are able to control their blood sugar through a combination of medication, weight loss, healthy eating, and exercise; others will eventually require insulin injections just like people with type 1.

THE GOOD NEWS

While there's no way to prevent type 1 diabetes, and you can't change certain type 2 risk factors, such as growing older or a family history of the disease, you can control other variables—namely, how much you exercise and what and how much you eat. Diet and lifestyle are so powerful that overweight people at risk for this disease can reduce their odds by simply losing 5–7 percent of their body weight. That's just 8–11 pounds for a 150-pound woman.

SUPER NUTRIENTS AND POWER FOODS
LEAN PROTEIN

What It Is: Protein helps build all of the cells and tissues in your body, from your red blood cells to your muscles. Your body also uses this nutrient to make enzymes, hormones, and even antibodies that fight off infection. However, some foods that are rich in protein, such as many cuts of red meat and full-fat milk and cheese, can also be high in fat and calories. Your better bet: lean, lower-calorie protein from poultry, fish, beans, soy foods (edamame, tofu), and lowfat dairy.

How It Balances Blood Sugar: Protein controls your appetite—specifically, it regulates hormones that tell your stomach to empty more slowly, so you feel fuller. It can even help you eat 10–20 percent fewer calories at your next meal or snack. Even if you're not trying to lose weight, that can prevent extra pounds from sneaking up as you get older. Aim for about 20 grams at each meal.

➤ **FACT** Protein takes up to six times more energy to digest than carbs or fat.

➤ **SMART TIP** Replacing some carbohydrates with protein can help shrink belly fat that's linked to insulin resistance. To learn how, check out the low-carb meal plan on page 232 in chapter 9.

➤ **GOOD TO KNOW!** Too much protein can put a strain on your kidneys, so limit your protein to no more than 100 grams a day. That's the equivalent of three small grilled boneless chicken breasts (a small chicken breast is about the size of a deck of cards).

WHY PEOPLE DON'T KNOW THEY HAVE DIABETES

Of the 29 million Americans who have diabetes, one-quarter of them don't even realize it, and another 86 million are hovering on the brink with its precursor, prediabetes. How can that be? Not everybody has the telltale symptoms of excessive thirst, fatigue, hunger, and a frequent need to urinate, so the early warning signs can be easy to brush off. But you shouldn't. In addition to the immediate danger of too much sugar in your bloodstream, which can be potentially fatal, having diabetes dramatically heightens your risk for other ills, including:

◆ Heart disease
◆ Stroke
◆ Blindness
◆ Pregnancy difficulties
◆ Kidney disease
◆ Nerve damage

Where to Find It:
NONFAT PLAIN GREEK YOGURT
With an impressive 17 grams of protein per 6-ounce container, Greek yogurt is one of the quickest, easiest ways to get your lean protein fix. When Dutch researchers fed volunteers either a high-carb or a high-protein yogurt breakfast, they noticed some curious differences in their subjects' hunger hormones afterward. Those who downed the protein-packed meal produced less ghrelin, a hormone that your stomach secretes to tell you it's time to eat—the less ghrelin you make, the better. At the same time, the volunteers in the study produced more cholecystokinin, a gut hormone that tells your digestive system to slow down, causing your stomach to empty more gradually.

➤ **QUICK IDEAS** Stir a couple of tablespoons of nonfat plain Greek yogurt into guacamole or hummus for a protein boost. It's also a great stand-in for mayo in deviled eggs or sour cream on a baked potato.

➤ **BONUS!** One 6-ounce container of nonfat plain Greek yogurt gives you nearly 20 percent of your daily calcium quota for strong bones and lower blood pressure.

PORK TENDERLOIN

When it comes to meat, there can be big differences in artery-clogging saturated fat. Take a rib eye steak, for example. One small 4-ounce serving dishes up 28 grams of protein. But along with that protein comes 18 grams of fat, of which six are saturated, as well as 279 calories. Have a similar-sized serving of pork tenderloin, and you'll get 30 grams of protein with 4 grams of total fat and only 1 ½ grams of saturated fat, at a slimming 162 calories.

➤ QUICK IDEA For a healthier version of fried rice, dice leftover pork tenderloin and toss with brown rice, edamame, light soy sauce, sliced scallions, and water chestnuts.

➤ BONUS! Pork tenderloin is an excellent source of niacin, a B vitamin that your body uses to convert food to energy.

UNDERSTANDING YOUR BLOOD SUGAR NUMBERS

A fasting blood glucose test can reveal if your blood sugar is normal, if you're pre-diabetic, or if you've already developed diabetes. Here's what the figures mean:

CATEGORY	FASTING BLOOD GLUCOSE*
Normal	70-99
Prediabetes	100-125
Diabetes	over 126

**In mg/dL, or milligrams per deciliter

TURKEY CUTLETS

Even though any kind of protein helps you burn a few extra calories, digesting protein from animal sources like chicken, pork, or beef uses more calories than eating vegetable protein from, say, beans or tofu. Skinless poultry is the leanest protein per ounce, followed by pork tenderloin, then steak. If you're already eating plenty of skinless, boneless chicken breasts, why not try turkey cutlets? At 34 grams of lean protein, they're only 167 calories and 2 grams of fat—with less than 1 gram of saturated fat—per 4-ounce cutlet, cooked.

➤ GOOD TO KNOW! Free-range turkeys are allowed to roam outside rather than being cooped up in a cage. While this may be a more humane way to raise turkeys, it doesn't affect their taste or nutrition.

➤ BONUS! Turkey is rich in zinc, a mineral that helps keep your immune system healthy and your fingernails strong.

Spot hidden sugars in food

Even seemingly healthy foods can be packed with stealth sugars. This quick cheat sheet shows where hidden sugars are lurking in foods that could be in your kitchen right now. One note: Food labels list sugar in grams. To convert grams to teaspoons simply divide by 4.

FOOD	TEASPOONS SUGAR
Ketchup (1 tablespoon)	1
Reduced fat French dressing (2 tablespoons)	1 ¼
Beef hot dog (1)	1 ½
BBQ sauce (1 tablespoon)	1 ½
Marinara sauce (½ cup)	1 ¾
Baked beans (½ cup)	2 ½
Maple brown sugar instant oatmeal (1 packet)	3
Rice milk (1 cup)	3
Agave (1 tablespoon)	3 ½
Granola (½ cup)	3 ½
Canned cranberry sauce (¼ cup)	5 ½

RECIPE

◆ Turkey Cutlets Piccata, page 208

MAGNESIUM

What It Is: Magnesium is one of those nutrients that never seems to get the credit it deserves. This mineral is so important that it's used in more than 300 chemical reactions in your body, helping to regulate heartbeat and blood pressure, keeping your bones and teeth strong, and aiding with muscle contractions.

How It Balances Blood Sugar: Magnesium helps your body use insulin—and ultimately glucose—efficiently. However, up to a quarter of people with diabetes have low magnesium levels. Here's why: with diabetes, excess glucose can build up in your blood stream. To rid the body of that extra sugar, your kidneys increase their production of urine. When they do, you lose sugar *and* flush out needed magnesium.

In a given day, most women attain only about 83 percent of the recommended 320 milligrams. As you get older, it's even more important to have magnesium on your radar, since you absorb less of it from food yet excrete more of it in your urine. If you're wondering if a supplement might help, keep in mind that popping magnesium pills can cause stomach woes ranging from nausea and cramps to diarrhea. So stick with magnesium-rich foods instead.

➤ DID YOU KNOW? Twelve to 18 percent of people with diabetes struggle with depression, compared to just 5–10 percent of nondiabetics. And a 2012 *Nutrition Journal* study found that the less magnesium in a diabetic person's diet, the more likely she is to battle the blues.

➤ FACT The best place to get magnesium is from plant foods such as green vegetables (think spinach and Swiss chard) as well as beans, nuts, seeds, and whole grains.

➤ GOOD TO KNOW! People who take certain medications known as proton pump inhibitors for acid reflux for longer than a year are more likely to be magnesium deficient. If you've been taking these long-term, talk to your doctor about how they may impact your magnesium levels.

Where to Find It:
BROWN RICE

How to have your favorite rice bowl *without* having your blood sugar soar: Simply swap in brown rice for white. Why? White rice is highly processed, which robs it of important nutrients like magnesium and fiber that normally slow digestion and the release of sugars into your bloodstream. In fact, brown rice supplies nearly four and a half times more magnesium than white rice, with a hefty 26 percent of your day's worth per cooked cup.

Another brown rice benefit: It has a lower glycemic index than its color-free sibling. Glycemic index (GI) is a measure of how quickly a food causes your blood sugar to rise. Stripped bare of bran and germ, white rice is rapidly digested, so it ranks high on the scale with a GI of 72 (or higher) out of a possible 100. Brown rice, which is left whole, has a lower GI of 48–62.

➤ QUICK IDEA Toss ½ cup of brown rice into a lunchtime salad to feel satisfied for hours.

➤ BONUS! One cup of cooked brown rice provides 5 grams of blood-sugar-leveling protein.

ONE MORE PLACE TO HUNT!

Look for grains that have the Whole Grains Council's Whole Grain Stamp on the package. And aim for foods containing at least 16 grams of whole grains per serving, or one-third of the recommended 48-gram daily goal.

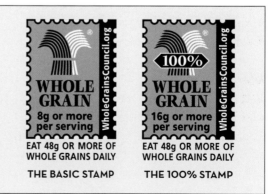

WHOLE GRAIN
8g or more per serving
WholeGrainsCouncil.org
EAT 48g OR MORE OF WHOLE GRAINS DAILY
THE BASIC STAMP

100%
WHOLE GRAIN
16g or more per serving
WholeGrainsCouncil.org
EAT 48g OR MORE OF WHOLE GRAINS DAILY
THE 100% STAMP

Carbohydrates

Don't get bogged down with total carbohydrates—how many carbs are in a food—as it doesn't distinguish between complex and refined carbs.

Since complex carbs and dietary fiber are often found together in food, the dietary fiber figure can be a helpful hint about carb quality. But just because a food has plenty of fiber doesn't always mean it contains healthy carbs. That's because some food companies fortify less-than-virtuous foods with added fiber. To figure it out, scan the ingredient list for filler fibers such as cellulose, hemicellulose, inulin, or chicory root, which lack the other nutrients you'd get from complex carbs.

The ingredient list can tell you the most about whether a food contains whole grains. Since ingredients are listed in order from greatest to least, look for any of these whole grains at the beginning of the ingredient list:

◆ Amaranth
◆ Barley
◆ Brown rice
◆ Buckwheat
◆ Bulgur
◆ Corn (not corn syrup)
◆ Farro
◆ Kamut
◆ Millet
◆ Oats or oatmeal
◆ Quinoa
◆ Rye
◆ Spelt
◆ Whole wheat
◆ Wheat berries

RECIPES
- Brown Rice Edamame Salad, page 151
- Cashew-Chicken Stir-Fry, page 164
- Chicken Vegetable Skewers, page 170
- Mexican Burrito Bowl, page 188

WHOLE GRAINS

What They Are: Technically more of a super *ingredient* than a single nutrient, a whole grain is any grain that has been minimally processed and still contains all three of its original parts, which are:

◆ **Bran** The grain's outermost layer; it's loaded with B vitamins, fiber, and antioxidants.

◆ **Germ** This is the plant's embryo. Like the bran, it's rich in B vitamins. The germ also provides protein and beneficial mono- and polyunsaturated fats.

◆ **Endosperm** Supplying protein and ample carbohydrates, this is the plant's food supply and the biggest part of the grain.

How They Balance Blood Sugar: Despite what you may have heard, carbs are not the enemy. In fact, carbohydrates can absolutely be part of a blood-sugar-friendly diet, provided they're the right kind. Rule of thumb: eat more complex carbohydrates from whole foods, and limit refined carbs from processed ones (you can read more about complex carbs on page 68 in chapter 5). Topping the list of good, complex carbs are whole grains, which work in multiple ways to prevent blood-sugar problems. You may already be getting them from bran cereal, oatmeal, brown rice, and whole-wheat bread and pasta. But there are loads of others, including barley, bulgur, millet, quinoa, and even popcorn.

Rich in slowly digested fiber, whole grains reduce the rate that you digest and absorb carbohydrates. That keeps you full and satisfied, helping you eat less and ultimately stay slimmer. However, whole grains aren't just about fiber. They're filled with nutrients that balance blood sugar, such as vitamins, minerals, and phytochemicals, potent plant substances that help fight disease.

➤ FACT Whole grains are so powerful that people who eat three to five servings of whole grains a day are 26 percent less likely to develop type 2 diabetes.

➤ GOOD TO KNOW! Health experts recommend making half your grains whole grains.

Where to Find Them:
BULGUR

Only about 5 percent of people make half of their grains each day whole grains. Maybe that's why 84 percent of Americans don't eat their daily allotment of 25 grams of fiber. Foods like bran flakes, brown rice, and whole wheat bread can help fill the void, but to really up your intake of high-quality whole grains, you'll need variety, and lots of it. Meet bulgur.

It's one of the most versatile yet underrated grains around. Plus, this Middle Eastern staple is only 151 calories per fluffy cooked cup.

➤ QUICK IDEA Turn bulgur into a main dish salad with chickpeas, tomatoes, cucumbers, and fresh mint.

➤ SMART TIP You can use cooked bulgur to cut down on red meat by folding it into burgers or meatloaf.

➤ GOOD TO KNOW! With 8 grams of fiber per cooked cup, bulgur gives you more roughage than practically any other grain.

➤ BONUS! A cup of cooked bulgur provides 6 grams of protein, which helps with blood-sugar control.

RECIPES
◆ Beet Tabbouleh with Grilled Chicken, page 162
◆ Mediterranean Shrimp and Bulgur, page 184

OTHER POWER FOODS TO BALANCE BLOOD SUGAR
APPLES

How They Balance Blood Sugar: They're rich in fiber and quercetin.

Think fruit can't be part of a blood-sugar-friendly diet? Think again. Since whole fruit packs plenty of digestion-slowing fiber, its natural sugar trickles into your system rather than flooding it. This fruit also boasts plentiful antioxidants such as quercetin, which enhances insulin secretion. Just be sure to eat your apple with the skin on, as the skin has up to six times as much quercetin as the flesh.

➤ **FACT** Harvard School of Public Health researchers found that women who ate at least two servings of whole fruit a week, especially apples, grapes, and blueberries, were 23 percent less likely to develop type 2 diabetes than those who sampled fruit only once a month.

➤ **QUICK IDEA** For a no-guilt dessert, core a whole apple and sprinkle with cinnamon and nutmeg. Cover and bake in a 325°F oven for 45 minutes.

RECIPES
* Apple Spinach Salad, page 147
* Tuna Fennel Wrap, page 156

ASPARAGUS

How It Balances Blood Sugar: It's rich in antioxidants.

Eating your green vegetables does more than deliver loads of vitamins and minerals. Green vegetables like asparagus are packed with antioxidants, such as polyphenols, vitamin C, and beta-carotene, which fight inflammation stemming from weight gain. And because asparagus is rich in fiber (3 grams per cup) yet low in calories (just 27 per cup), it's ideal for filling your plate without expanding your waistline.

➤ **FACT** When British researchers reviewed the results of six studies, they found that downing about 5 ounces of green leafy vegetables a day (slightly less than 1 cup of asparagus) cut a person's chances of type 2 diabetes by 14 percent.

➤ **QUICK IDEA** Roasted asparagus makes a simple side dish. Simply toss a bunch of trimmed, cleaned asparagus with 1 tablespoon of olive oil; season with garlic powder, sea salt, and pepper; and roast on a baking sheet in a 400°F oven for 15 minutes.

RECIPES
* Lemon Pasta with Salmon and Asparagus, page 180
* Orange-Soy Tofu Stir-Fry, page 190
* Pasta with Asparagus, Cannellini, and Parmesan, page 185
* Pepper-Crusted Tuna with Sesame Asparagus, page 192

BLUEBERRIES

How They Balance Blood Sugar: They're rich in compounds that block carbohydrate absorption.

Hippocrates was on to something when he said, "Let food be thy medicine." Just as certain diabetes medications lower blood sugar by blocking the absorption of glucose in your intestine, so do certain compounds in blueberries. Blueberries also enhance insulin sensitivity. When scientists in a *Journal of Nutrition* study fed insulin-resistant

THINK BEFORE YOU DRINK!

Sipping just one or two sugary drinks a day has been linked to a 26 percent increase in your chance of developing diabetes.

volunteers a smoothie spiked with either freeze-dried blueberry powder or a placebo twice a day for 6 weeks, the blueberry group experienced a significant boost in insulin sensitivity.

➤ QUICK IDEAS Mix ½ cup of fresh or thawed frozen blueberries into your morning cereal, whole-wheat pancakes, or oatmeal. Or, for a flavor-packed side dish, try them in couscous or quinoa.

➤ GOOD TO KNOW! One cup of blueberries has 84 calories, about the same amount of fiber you'd get from 2 small slices of whole-wheat bread.

➤ BONUS! Antioxidant-rich blueberries are beneficial for heart and brain health and may protect against certain kinds of cancer.

———

RECIPES
◆ Better-for-You Blueberry Waffles, page 137
◆ Cantaloupe Breakfast Bowl, page 138

CHICKPEAS

How They Balance Blood Sugar: They're low on the glycemic index.

With a glycemic index of 33, chickpeas are one of the lowest GI foods around. Beyond that, they're filled with fiber and lean protein, making them a perfect food for keeping your blood sugar on an even keel. They're so effective that people who followed a diet that included at least 1 cup of beans a day, such as chickpeas, experienced a substantial drop in a blood sugar measurement known as HbA1C. Never heard of HbA1C? It reveals glucose levels over a three-month period. Doctors are increasingly using

---

LIQUID ASSETS
Coffee

———

Coffee does more than just wake you up in the morning. Research shows it can help forestall diabetes. A 2009 review of 18 different studies in the journal *Diabetology and Metabolic Syndrome* found that drinking 4 or more cups of coffee a day, supplying roughly 400 milligrams of caffeine, helped ward off type 2 diabetes. While that may sound like a hefty dose, it's really not much more than the 260 milligrams that most adults average in a day (or the amount you'd get from a 12-ounce "tall" Starbucks coffee). Plus, what qualifies as a "cup" of coffee in the lab is a tiny 6–8 ounces.

In terms of how caffeine works, experts suspect multiple mechanisms. On the simplest level, caffeine boosts your calorie burn and helps you feel full, so it may provide a slight weight-loss edge. But it's not all about caffeine. Coffee also contains more than a thousand different compounds that benefit blood sugar, including nutrients like magnesium and chlorogenic acid, which helps block the absorption of carbs. Meaning? Even decaf coffee may help.

HbA1C, along with fasting glucose, to gain a more accurate understanding of a person's long-term blood sugar health.

➤ QUICK IDEAS Mild-tasting chickpeas (also called garbanzo beans) are the ultimate convenience food. Simply pop open a can, rinse, and toss them into a salad, pasta, or soup. No soaking, cooking, or reheating required!

➤ **BONUS!** Chickpeas are a top source of manganese, a mineral that helps you metabolize carbs, protein, and fat. A cup provides two-thirds of your daily dose.

———

RECIPES

- ◆ Couscous with Chickpeas, page 151
- ◆ Curried Chickpea Pita, page 152
- ◆ Mediterranean Pasta Salad, page 153

CINNAMON

How It Balances Blood Sugar: It's rich in compounds that help you use insulin more efficiently.

Want to cut down on sugar without sacrificing sweetness? With only 6 calories per teaspoon, cinnamon can help. For thousands of years, the Chinese have used it to treat diabetes, and now a growing body of research finds it can help lower fasting glucose and HbA1C levels. Experts aren't sure exactly how it works, but they believe cinnamon may enhance insulin sensitivity and reduce the rate that your body absorbs carbs.

➤ **QUICK IDEA** Give your coffee a blood-sugar-balancing boost by sprinkling cinnamon into ground coffee before brewing.

➤ **BONUS!** Preliminary research indicates that cinnamon may lower blood pressure, cholesterol, and triglycerides.

THE TRUTH ABOUT
Artificial sweeteners

For years, people have been using artificial sweeteners to cut sugar and calories. Recently, however, sugar substitutes have come under the microscope, taking the blame for everything from cancer to heart disease to, ironically, weight gain. From a health perspective, these sweeteners have been on supermarket shelves for decades without any conclusive evidence that they cause cancer. As for heart disease? A tiny handful of studies made headlines linking diet soda to heart ills. But the research is so scant, it's unclear if the artificial sweeteners are to blame or if the diet soda drinkers have other habits (for instance, eating an unhealthy diet) that might be hurting their hearts.

Meanwhile, some studies have connected sugar substitutes to a bigger appetite and weight gain, and others have found that they can help people cut calories and drop pounds. Right now, both the American Diabetes Association and the American Heart Association agree that there's not enough research to say for sure.

➤ **BOTTOM LINE:** There's certainly no evidence that artificial sweeteners are worse for you than the empty calories that come from sugar-filled sodas, iced teas, and lattes, as well as candies and desserts—all of which can lead to obesity, heart disease, and diabetes. That said, a 16-calorie teaspoon of sugar every now and then probably won't hurt you either.

FLAXSEED

How It Balances Blood Sugar: It's rich in lignans.

Flaxseed is nature's number one source of lignans, plant chemicals that are believed to help your body use insulin more efficiently. Flax has an incredible 100 times more lignans than any other food. Plus, it's the number one source of the power lignan secoisolariciresinol diglucoside (try saying that 10 times fast!). This substance may keep prediabetes from snowballing into all-out diabetes by reducing inflammation and slowing the absorption of glucose from foods. And you don't need a lot of flax to do the trick. A 2013 *Nutrition Research* study found that adding just 2 tablespoons of ground flaxseed to meals daily for 3 months lowered insulin levels by 17 percent in prediabetic volunteers.

➤ **SMART TIP** If you haven't eaten flaxseed before, work it into your diet slowly. Because flaxseed is also a natural laxative, you'll want to give your digestive system a chance to adjust to it gradually.

➤ **FACT** A study in the journal *Diabetes Care* found that women with the most lignans in their diets were 36 percent less likely to develop type 2 diabetes.

NUTRITIONIST'S NOTE
On added sugars

When I was studying to become a dietitian, fat took the blame for everything from weight gain to heart disease. These days, many people are calling out sugar as the newest nutrition villain. But even though sugar is a huge source of empty calories, it's not necessary to eliminate it from your plate (or glass) entirely. More important? Figure out whether it's natural sugar found in whole foods, which can travel with important nutrients such as vitamins, minerals, and fiber; or empty-calorie added sugar from processed foods like candy, cookies, and soda. You can find out for sure by checking out the Nutrition facts panel on the food package, which will tell you exactly how much sugar is in a food and—more importantly—how much of it is added sugar.

➤ **QUICK IDEA** Sprinkle 1 tablespoon of flaxseed into your morning cereal or stir it into yogurt.

➤ **BONUS!** Lignans keep your bones strong, improve digestive health, and prevent heart disease.

GARLIC

How It Balances Blood Sugar: It's rich in antioxidants.

When diabetes takes hold, it doesn't just cause your blood sugar to skyrocket; your entire metabolism goes haywire. When it does, your body starts to generate harmful compounds known as free radicals, which attack and damage your cells through oxidation. If that weren't trouble enough, diabetes hands you a double whammy by causing your internal supply of antioxidants to plummet. With more free radicals, and fewer antioxidants to fight them, your cells' glucose-burning machinery becomes damaged, which leads to insulin resistance. Garlic to the rescue! It provides compounds that stomp out free radicals, resulting in less insulin resistance and better blood sugar.

➤ **QUICK IDEA** For a healthier version of garlic bread, slice off the top and bottom of a head of garlic, drizzle with olive oil, wrap in foil, and roast in a 400°F oven for 30 minutes. Unwrap, let cool slightly, and squeeze the inside of each garlic clove over sliced whole-wheat toast and spread like butter.

➤ **SMART TIP** A sign that garlic is past its prime?

HABIT REHAB
Nighttime noshing

Do you automatically curl up with a bag of chips or handful of cookies after dinner? Break that evening snacking cycle, and you'll stay lighter and leaner.

◆ **Start early.** Studies find that eating regular meals, beginning with breakfast, improves insulin sensitivity and helps you stay full throughout the day. For the most mileage, make sure your breakfast contains some lean protein from foods like eggs, Greek yogurt, or lowfat cottage cheese.

◆ **Keep it in the kitchen.** If you've eaten sensibly all day but still can't stop noshing at night, your problem could be habit, not hunger. Your goal: Make nighttime nibbling more difficult, and you'll be less likely to give in to it. That means snacking only at the kitchen table—with no TV, phone, computer, or tablet to distract you—and only eating off of a plate or out of a bowl.

◆ **Hit the relax button.** After a tough day, it's easy to want to drown your sorrows in a comforting pint of chocolate fudge brownie ice cream. But there is a better way. Rather than waiting for the day's stress to snowball after dinner, nip it in the bud. Try a late afternoon workout, walk, or yoga class. Or, if you can't spare the time, steal 5 or 10 quiet minutes before dinner for deep breathing or meditation.

◆ **Turn in early.** Would you believe that too little sleep could be fueling your nighttime cravings? A 2009 *American Journal of Clinical Nutrition* study says it's true. When volunteers were deprived of 2 hours of sleep a night, they took in 25 percent more snack calories the following evening (for more on how this happens see "Five Ways to Sleep Better Tonight" on page 41). Another benefit of hitting the hay early: If you're sleeping, you won't be snacking.

Loose skin. Instead, look for heads with tight skins. It may be harder to peel, but it's fresher.

➤ BONUS! Garlic is a potent cancer preventer. Chopping garlic 10 minutes before you use it allows even more cancer fighters known as organosulfur compounds to form.

PUMPKIN SEEDS

How They Balance Blood Sugar: They're rich in lignans and globulins.

Like flaxseed, pumpkin seeds, or pepitas, are prime sources of lignans, which help your body use insulin more efficiently. Used as an African folk remedy to treat diabetes, pepitas are also rich in globulins, special proteins that may lower blood sugar. Plus, pumpkin seeds can help trim your waistline. One quarter cup of seeds has 10 grams of protein and 2 grams of fiber for a modest 180 calories.

➤ QUICK IDEAS Pumpkin seeds aren't just for Halloween. Add them into trail mix, swap them in for nuts in pesto, or sprinkle them on top of soup, chili, or guacamole.

➤ SMART TIP Spray whole pumpkin seeds with olive oil cooking spray and sprinkle with cinnamon, curry powder, or cumin. Roast in a 300°F oven for 45 minutes.

➤ BONUS! Pumpkin seeds are a magnesium powerhouse with half your day's worth of this blood-sugar-balancing mineral per ¼ cup.

RECIPE

◆ Spicy Trail Mix, page 226

RED BELL PEPPERS

How They Balance Blood Sugar: They're rich in vitamin C.

FIVE WAYS TO SLEEP BETTER TONIGHT

Too little shuteye leaves you dragging the next day. It can also knock your hunger hormones off balance, which can cause extra weight to creep on. If you'd like to slumber more soundly, try these tips:

1 **Find a fresh laundry detergent.** New research shows that pleasant smells can help you drift off to sleep more easily, so start with your bedding. A National Sleep Foundation survey found that three-quarters of people said they slept better when their sheets had a clean smell.

2 **Unplug.** Ninety-five percent of people use electronics an hour before turning off the lights. Yet it's not the best idea. Blue light from computers and cell phones interferes with your body's production of melatonin, a hormone that normally helps lull you to sleep. If possible, banish all electronics from your bedroom. If not, unplug at least an hour before bedtime.

3 **Dim the lights.** Bright lights before bed also confuse your body. Relaxing in a dimly lit room the hour before you turn in can help you drift off faster.

4 **Keep it cool.** When you sleep, your body temperature naturally falls. You can help the process by turning the thermostat in your bedroom down to 65 degrees, the optimal temperature recommended by the National Sleep Foundation for a sound night's sleep.

5 **Drown out distractions.** Rattling pipes, barking dogs, snoring spouses, and honking horns can all make you toss and turn. Muffle them with white noise, the kind of generic, monotonous sound made by a fan or air conditioner. In the winter, try a white-noise machine.

Prediabetes and diabetes can take a toll on your heart health. The less steady your blood sugar, the worse free-radical-related blood-vessel damage becomes. Enter vitamin C, which has been found to protect your vessels from that type of harm. At only 37 calories, one sliced red bell pepper gives you two times the vitamin C you need in a day (75 milligrams).

➤ **GOOD TO KNOW!** One orange, 1 cup of strawberries, or one kiwi also provide your daily allowance of C.

➤ **BONUS!** Red bell peppers are rich in vitamin A for healthy skin and a strong immune system. One pepper provides more than a quarter of your day's worth.

RECIPES

- Breakfast Burrito, page 138
- Orange-Soy Tofu Stir-Fry, page 190
- Slow Cooker Italian Lentil and Vegetable Stew, page 199

VINEGAR

How It Balances Blood Sugar: It's rich in acetic acid.

Vinegar contains acetic acid, a secret weapon in the fight against diabetes. To find out just how effective acetic acid is at regulating blood sugar, Swedish researchers fed volunteers white bread soaked in vinegar with varying levels of acetic acid. The more acetic acid each meal contained, the more effectively it lowered blood sugar and insulin levels, and the better it was at keeping volunteers full. Experts aren't sure exactly why acetic acid is such strong medicine, but they suspect it slows the release of food from your stomach. It also works in your gut to reduce the activity of enzymes that break down certain sugars, so the sugars enter your system more gradually.

➤ **QUICK IDEA** Skip the mayo on your sandwich, and drizzle it with a little olive oil and red wine vinegar instead.

➤ **SMART TIP** The easiest way to eat more acetic acid is by tossing your salad with vinaigrette, but you can also find it in pickles and fermented foods like sauerkraut.

➤ **GOOD TO KNOW!** Even though red wine, distilled, and cider vinegars are nearly calorie-free, balsamic contains 15 calories per tablespoon.

CHECKLIST
For balanced blood sugar

○ Maintaining a healthy body weight is one of the best ways to reduce your risk of diabetes. If you have a few pounds to lose, aim for about 1,500 calories a day. The meal plan in this chapter can show you how.

○ Take a few minutes to pencil in 30 minutes of brisk walking, biking, hiking, or swimming on your calendar on most days. For busy days when you can't commit to a full 30 minutes at once, three 10-minute walks can do the trick.

○ A good night's sleep can help control your appetite, not to mention give you more energy, so aim for at least 7 hours of shut-eye a night.

○ Don't forget to read the ingredient list to spot added sugars in foods.

○ Aim to make at least half your daily grains whole. Top choices include barley, bulgur, brown rice, quinoa, and whole-wheat bread, couscous, and pasta.

○ Eating lean protein with every meal will help control your appetite and keep your blood sugar on an even keel. Lowfat milk, Greek yogurt, eggs, chicken, pork tenderloin, turkey, and fish are your best picks.

○ Try to get enough magnesium each day by eating plenty of green vegetables, whole grains, and beans.

○ For more blood-sugar-balancing lignans, snack on nuts and pumpkin seeds, or sprinkle flaxseed into oatmeal, cold cereal, or yogurt.

○ Remember, antioxidants and vitamin C can also improve blood sugar, so be sure to eat at least five servings of fruits and vegetables a day.

One-week meal plan for balanced blood sugar

	BREAKFAST	LUNCH	DINNER
DAY 1	Tropical Greek Yogurt Breakfast Parfait*	Black Bean Burger Salad*	Pasta with Asparagus, Cannellini, and Parmesan*
DAY 2	Better-for-You Blueberry Waffles*	Apple Spinach Salad*	Greek-Style Tilapia* 1 cup microwaved frozen peas tossed with 2 teaspoons olive oil
DAY 3	Spinach-Feta Omelet* ½ grapefruit	Brown Rice Edamame Salad*	Beet Tabbouleh with Grilled Chicken* Salad of ½ romaine lettuce heart and 2 large slices tomato drizzled with 1 teaspoon extra virgin olive oil and 1 teaspoon balsamic vinegar
DAY 4	1 slice whole wheat toast, topped with 2 tablespoons nut butter and 1 sliced apple	Asian Chicken Tacos*	Mediterranean Shrimp and Bulgur* 1 cup sliced strawberries drizzled with 1 tablespoon balsamic vinegar
DAY 5	Crunchy Sunflower Butter Sandwich*	Couscous with Chickpeas*	Turkey Cutlets Piccata* 2 cups baby spinach sautéed in 1 teaspoon olive oil ¼ cup brown rice, prepared according to package directions
DAY 6	Avocado Swiss Breakfast Sandwich*	Salmon Pesto Sandwich* ¼ cup rinsed and drained no-salt-added canned chickpeas with 1 cup sliced grape tomatoes and 1 teaspoon balsamic vinegar	Apricot Roast Pork Medallions* 1 medium baked sweet potato
DAY 7	Breakfast Burrito*	BBQ Turkey Burger* 10 steamed asparagus spears with 2 teaspoons balsamic vinegar	Mediterranean Steak Salad*

*Recipe included in chapter 9

Chia Pudding*

1 hardboiled egg sprinkled with celery salt + 1 orange

---

1 nut-based snack bar

1 piece reduced-fat string cheese + 1 pear

Chocolate Chili Popcorn*

1 sliced bell pepper dipped in 1/4 cup hummus

Spicy Trail Mix*

1/4 cup part-skim ricotta mixed with 1 large pinch cinnamon on 8 small whole-wheat crackers

---

6 ounces nonfat plain Greek yogurt with 1/2 cup blueberries

12-ounce nonfat latte (6 ounces nonfat milk warmed in the microwave + 6 ounces hot brewed coffee) + 3/4 cup grapes

---

1 cup cubed cantaloupe + 25 pistachio nuts

Unlimited vegetables dipped in 3/4 cup plain yogurt mixed with a large pinch curry powder

---

1 apple and 2 1-inch Brie cubes

3/4 cup edamame

CHAPTER 4

Keep Cancer at Bay

Cancer strikes one out of three women, but adopting healthier habits today can cut your risk by a third. Powerful prevention is eating a nutritious, produce-rich diet.

HOW CANCER DEVELOPS

Did you know that cancer isn't just one disease? It's actually about 100 different diseases, all caused by abnormal cell growth, and most are named for the organ or area of the body they affect. It starts in your DNA, which is like your cells' genetic command center, responsible for everything from deciding your hair color to telling your cells how quickly and accurately to divide. However, factors like pollution, infections, smoking, UV light, and certain substances in the food you eat can all damage your DNA. If that happens once in a while, it's no big deal. Your cells are equipped with their own built-in DNA repair system to help overcome the occasional injury. But when those stresses happen over and over, it can cause mutations to occur, which change

you can take to stay cancer-free. The first? Keeping an eye on the scale, as one-third of cancers are linked to lifestyle factors such as excess body fat, lack of exercise, and poor nutrition. As discussed in chapter 3, fat can boost the production of diabetes-causing compounds. Well, it also increases hormones and proteins that favor cancer formation.

In this chapter, you'll learn how loading up on certain Power Foods—primarily plant foods like fruits, vegetables, beans, nuts, seeds, and whole grains—can shore up your anticancer defenses. They're all filled with antioxidants, as well as compounds known as phytonutrients that safeguard and repair DNA (for more on phytonutrients, turn to page 22 in chapter 2). By making these the foundation of your diet, you'll always have a steady stream of protection on tap. That doesn't mean you have to give up meat, chicken, fish, or dairy. You just want to think of them as accents to a plant-forward diet. And eating this way doesn't simply build your body's anticancer arsenal. Paired with smart portion sizes, it practically guarantees weight loss—a win-win.

➤ SMART TIP Other ways to reduce your

the rate at which cells reproduce, divide, and even die. That, in turn, can cause damaged cells to grow out of control and form tumors or infiltrate your bloodstream. Because this damage can take years or even decades to develop, the older you are, the more cancer-prone you become.

THE GOOD NEWS

You may not be able to completely protect your DNA from harm, but there are steps

THE ALCOHOL-CANCER CONNECTION

Sure, alcohol can help your heart, but it's important to keep tabs on those cocktails. Like tobacco, alcohol is a carcinogen—its ethanol disrupts your DNA. So the more you drink, the greater your chances of developing liver, breast, and colon cancer, to name a few. That's why the American Cancer Society recommends that women limit alcohol to no more than one drink a day. If you're concerned about breast cancer, you may want to be even more mindful, as just three drinks a week can bump up your breast cancer risk by 15 percent.

cancer risk: choosing not to smoke, and wearing protection whenever you're in the sun.

SUPER NUTRIENTS AND POWER FOODS
FIBER

What It Is: As you may remember from chapter 2, there are two main forms of fiber: soluble fiber, from fruits, vegetables, beans, nuts, seeds, and some whole grains like oats and barley, and insoluble fiber, from whole-wheat foods. You can't digest any type of fiber, but it still passes along amazing health benefits such as keeping you regular, lowering cholesterol, stabilizing blood sugar, and guarding against cancer.

How It Fights Cancer: Fiber works in several different ways to reduce your odds of certain cancers, especially colorectal cancer. On the most basic level, fiber expands in your gut like a sponge so it helps you stay full. And when you're more satisfied, you're less likely to overeat and gain weight. But the real magic happens in your colon, where fiber works like a broom, moving things along so harmful waste products don't have the opportunity to accumulate and cause harm.

Fiber also thwarts cancer by encouraging the growth of healthy bacteria in your colon. Your colon is like a gigantic petri dish that's home to more than 400 species of bacteria, some of which are helpful and others of which are not so much. Because the beneficial bacteria nourish your colon and fight cancer-causing inflammation, it's important to keep them happy and thriving. Special kinds of fiber, known as prebiotics, can do

NUTRITIONIST'S NOTE
On fiber

Nutrition experts recommend consuming at least 25 grams of fiber a day, which can sound like a tall order. So, many of my clients ask about foods like double-fiber bread or bran cereal with added fiber. What I tell them is that getting the optimal amount of roughage isn't about loading up on one or two foods with unnatural amounts of added fiber at one (or two) meals a day. A better strategy? Eat smaller amounts of naturally fiber-rich foods throughout the day. It's easier on your digestive system. Plus, including fiber at every meal means it regulates blood sugar, keeps you full, and lowers cholesterol throughout the day. A final benefit of whole fiber-filled foods is that they're almost always packed with other nutrients, such as vitamins, minerals, healthy fats, phytonutrients, and antioxidants. Fill your plate with quality, minimally processed fruits, vegetables, whole grains, nuts, seeds, and beans, and the quantity will follow.

this. You can get them from foods like whole-wheat bread and cereal, bananas, artichokes, and chicory root. After you eat prebiotics, they travel to your colon, where they're fermented. That process of fermentation produces powerful substances known as short-chain fatty acids, which nourish colon cells, helping them stay healthy and cancer-free.

ALL ABOARD!
Help your family eat more produce

If it seems like your family lets out a collective groan every time you tell them to eat their fruits and vegetables, you have a lot of company. Roughly a third of adults and teens say they eat fruits and vegetables less than once a day. Here are seven simple (and sometimes sneaky) ways to entice your family to eat more fruits and vegetables:

1 Put them where they can see them. If you expect your kids to go rummaging through the produce drawer for a piece of fruit, it's not going to happen. Instead, why not put a big bowl of fruit on the countertop so they can grab some as they go by? Try serving something they can scoop up by the handful, like grapes or berries, for after school or on the weekend.

2 Make it easy on yourself. Raw vegetables often have just as much nutrition as cooked. So, if your family is happy to munch on baby carrots and sliced bell peppers, don't worry about doing more. And since most kids (and spouses) will eat salad, keep a bag of prewashed lettuce in your fridge for a quick side.

3 Don't overthink it. You may have heard that carrots and beets are overflowing with sugar, or that potatoes and corn don't count because they're high in carbs. Forget it all. They're vegetables. If your family will eat them, put them on the table.

4 Accessorize. Maybe your brood won't eat straight-up asparagus. But what if it was topped with some pecorino and lemon zest? A little adornment can go a long way in converting lukewarm vegetable eaters into all-out fans. Try sprinkling sunflower or pumpkin seeds over salads; toss broccoli with pine nuts, garlic, and olive oil; or crumble goat cheese over roasted squash. Or spoon a healthy tomato sauce over scrambled eggs, grilled chicken breasts, or baked potatoes.

5 Use some camouflage. You don't need to hide your family's vegetables, but it can help to disguise them just a tad. Stir some drained, rinsed canned beans into chili, dump them into soup, or tuck them into quesadillas. The same works for frozen corn.

6 Don't forget dessert. No need to feel guilty about dessert when it's fruit-filled. In spring and summer, grill pineapple, peaches, or plums for a warm, gooey treat. During the colder months, whip up Roasted Pears (you'll find the recipe on page 219), or serve sliced pears or apples sprinkled with a little Gorgonzola cheese and walnuts.

Another reason to eat more fiber is that it may protect against breast cancer. A recent *Annals of Oncology* review of 16 studies found that for every 10 grams of daily fiber a woman eats, her breast cancer odds drop by 5 percent, particularly if she consumes 25 grams a day or more. One reason may be fiber's ability to lower estrogen, a hormone that can encourage breast cancer development. When a woman eats fiber, especially the soluble kinds found in oats, barley, peas, beans, and lentils, it binds to estrogens, ferrying them out of the body. With fewer available estrogens, breast cancer is less likely to occur.

Where to Find It:
PEAS

Peas are unique in that they're a vegetable as well as a legume, a plant that grows in a pod (e.g., chickpeas, black beans, soybeans, and lentils). Just like their bean cousins, peas are packed with fiber, with 7 grams per cup. Frozen peas receive high marks for convenience. They won't spoil, and there's no washing, chopping, or trimming. Plus, you can microwave them in a flash (for an instant side dish, simply drizzle them with a little olive oil).

➤ FACT Peas are rich in coumestrol, a plant compound that prevents stomach cancer. When Mexican researchers interviewed over 700 people about their diets, they found that those who downed the most coumestrol from foods like peas and beans were a third less likely to develop stomach cancer.

➤ QUICK IDEA Pump up fiber by stirring peas into macaroni and cheese or whole-wheat pasta with your favorite marinara sauce.

FOOD LABEL SLEUTH
Cereal

Dense cereals (like granola) pack loads of calories into a very small serving. So take a close look at the serving size before you pour. If it's only ¼ or ½ cup, it's going to be hard to stick with just one serving. Instead, seek out cereals with a serving size of about 1 cup and no more than 200 calories per serving.

Your morning meal is your best opportunity to squeeze fiber into the day, so look for cereals with roughly 5–8 grams per serving. Sound like a lot? Keep in mind that your daily goal is at least 25 grams.

Remember, every 4 grams of added sugar equals 1 teaspoon. While there's no hard and fast rule, consider 8 grams, or 2 teaspoons, a reasonable cap.

Have you ever noticed how the Nutrition Facts panel on some cereal boxes seems to go on forever? Don't be reeled in by the exhaustive list of added vitamins and minerals. If your diet is healthy, you're likely getting plenty of these already.

Check the ingredients list for the word "whole," as in whole wheat or whole oats or for other power grains like brown rice or spelt (find a full list of whole grains in the "Food Label Sleuth: Carbohydrates" on page 34 in chapter 3). A bonus? Seeds. Fiber-rich flax, hemp, chia, sunflower, and pumpkin are all winners.

CAN A VIRUS CAUSE CANCER?

It may be hard to believe, but 15 percent of cancers are caused by viruses like HPV (the human papillomavirus) or hepatitis B or C. How's that? When you become sick with a virus or bacterial infection, your body fights back by releasing immune cells that are programmed to battle foreign invaders. Even though that's a good thing, those defenses can sometimes inadvertently hit surrounding cells, injuring their DNA. When inflammation from viruses becomes chronic, it may be hard for your cells to repair the damage. That's where flavonoids come in. They make inflammation less likely to cause long-term harm to your cells.

➤ **BONUS!** One cup of cooked peas gives you 8 grams of protein.

RECIPE
◆ Curried Rice with Shrimp and Peas, page 171

POMEGRANATES

Beyond whole grains and beans, fruits with seeds—like raspberries, strawberries, black-berries, and pomegranates—are great ways to rack up extra fiber. One cup of pomegranate seeds (also called arils) gives you 7 grams of roughage. And fiber isn't the only way pome-granates help thwart cancer. These ruby fruits are also rich in ellagitannins, compounds that prevent tumors from growing. How so? When a tumor grows, it can develop its own blood supply, which feeds and nourishes it. Ellagi-tannins help prevent that blood supply from ever developing in the first place.

➤ **GOOD TO KNOW!** In addition to pomegran-ates, you can find ellagitannins in strawber-ries, raspberries, walnuts, and almonds.

➤ **QUICK IDEA** Toss pomegranate seeds into a baby spinach, romaine, or kale salad with

sliced pears for an instant fiber boost.

RECIPE
◆ Pomegranate-Apricot Breakfast Crostini, page 143

FLAVONOIDS

What They Are: Found in all kinds of plant foods, flavonoids are an enormous family of more than 4,000 different antioxidant plant chemicals that scavenge up the free radicals that can harm your DNA.

How They Fight Cancer: Flavonoids regulate genes that control the rate that your cells grow and reproduce. Imagine your genes are a light switch. When you flip the switch on, cells divide and multi-ply. Turn it off, and they stop growing. And, where cancer is involved, the "off" part of the equation is as important as the "on" part. While your cells have mechanisms to repair occasional DNA damage, speedy cell growth can cause mutations to occur so quickly that your cells don't have a chance to mend the injury. Once those mutated cells start growing, cancers form. Flavonoids keep things on track by controlling those on and off switches, ensuring that cells reproduce slowly and methodically.

➤ GOOD TO KNOW! Top sources of flavonoids include berries, red grapes, tea, chocolate, citrus fruits, and apples.

Where to Find Them:
GRAPEFRUIT

This citrus fruit guards against cancer in two ways. First, it contains limonin, a flavonoid that lowers the level of an inflammation-causing substance that's been linked to colon cancer. Grapefruit may cut your cancer odds by helping you stay slimmer as well. When researchers fed obese volunteers either half a grapefruit or a placebo before meals for 3 months, the grapefruit group lost 3.5 pounds compared to 0.66 pound for their counterparts who popped a placebo. Why? At just 50 calories per half, grapefruit is a good source of filling fiber (2 grams) plus it's rich in vitamin C (75 percent of your daily recommendation).

➤ BONUS! Grapefruit helps reduce cholesterol. People who added one grapefruit a day to their diet for a month lowered their total and LDL cholesterol up to 16 and 20 percent respectively (read more about LDL on page 11 in chapter 2).

➤ SMART TIP Grapefruit can interfere with the metabolism of certain medications, especially statins to lower cholesterol and calcium-channel blockers for high blood pressure. If you're on prescription medication, speak with your doctor before adding grapefruit to your diet.

RECIPE
◆ Grilled Chicken Salad with Avocado and Grapefruit, page 178

SHALLOTS

Move over, onions! When matched against ten different varieties of onions in a Cornell University study, shallots beat every single onion hands-down in terms of total antioxidant content. And that's not all. Shallots also contain special flavonoids known as phenolic compounds that prevent free radicals from attacking your DNA. Swap in shallots for Vidalia onions, and you'll rack up six times more of these cancer fighters.

➤ GOOD TO KNOW! Flavor-wise, these little bulbs taste like a cross between garlic and onions, so they're more mellow than your average onion.

➤ BONUS! Shallots are loaded with quercetin, a flavonoid that keeps insulin on an even keel.

➤ QUICK IDEAS Whisk chopped shallots into your favorite vinaigrette, swap them for sautéed onions in your next risotto, or sauté them in olive oil and tuck them into an omelet.

➤ SMART TIP To chop a shallot, first cut off the stem. Then remove the peel with a paring knife. Finally, cut the shallot in half, cut off the root, and then slice or chop.

RECIPES
◆ Cumin-Spiced Pumpkin Soup, page 217
◆ Slow Cooker Butternut Squash Barley Risotto, page 197

TOFU

Soy foods like tofu may lower your risk for hormone-sensitive cancers, especially breast cancer. One reason is the special flavonoids in soy known as isoflavones. Isoflavones are phytoestrogens, plant substances that are similar in structure to estrogen. This likeness gives isoflavones the ability to act like estrogen or to block its action—a good thing, as too much estrogen can fuel the growth of breast, endometrial, and uterine cancers. Mild in taste, tofu is an unbelievably versatile soybean-based curd.

➤ QUICK IDEAS What to do with tofu? Slice it and sear it like a steak, dice it and toss it into stir-fries, or even purée it for soups, smoothies, and sauces.

➤ GOOD TO KNOW! Isoflavone supplements don't protect against breast cancer; however, diets rich in whole soy foods such as tofu, edamame, and soymilk do.

➤ BONUS! Soy has been linked to better heart and brain health.

➤ FACT Women in Asian nations who traditionally eat lots of whole soy foods are more than three times less likely to develop breast cancer than their Western counterparts.

➤ DID YOU KNOW? Soy provides the same kind of complete high-quality protein that you'd get from meat, poultry, fish, eggs, and dairy.

RECIPE
◆ Orange-Soy Tofu Stir-Fry, page 190

GLUCOSINOLATES

What They Are: Flavonoids aren't the only plant chemicals that combat cancer. Glucosinolates are unique substances found only in cruciferous vegetables such as broccoli and kale. In addition to fighting cancer, they give these vegetables their characteristic bitter flavor.

How They Fight Cancer: Ask someone to name the best vegetable to fight cancer and, chances are, they'll say broccoli. The answer has to do with broccoli's glucosinolates. After you eat a cruciferous vegetable, such as broccoli, your body breaks its glucosinolates down into indoles and isothiocyanates, powerful scavengers that whisk carcinogens out of your body. These substances also encourage a process known as apoptosis, a critical cancer-defense mechanism in which cells self-destruct when they're damaged.

LIQUID ASSETS
Green tea

All tea is made from the leaves of the *Camellia sinensis* plant. Unlike black or oolong tea leaves, which are crushed and heated, green tea leaves are steamed, leaving more of their cancer-combating flavonoids intact—particularly one called epigallocatechin-3-gallate (ECGG). For a long time, experts have known that ECGG is an incredibly powerful antioxidant. Now, they're learning that it may protect against cancer by homing in on a protein known as HSP90, which is believed to kick off the first steps in the cancer process. What's more, green tea is calorie-free, and drinking 3 cups a day has been shown to reduce your heart-attack risk. So sip to your heart's content!

THE TRUTH ABOUT
Detox diets and cleanses

Have you tried—or thought about trying—a detox diet or a cleanse to drop a few quick pounds? Or maybe you've heard these can rid your body of carcinogens? Don't waste your time and money. Your cells already have their own natural defense system that scavenges and disables noxious free radicals and carcinogens. Beyond that, since old cells are more prone to errors, your cells are constantly turning over and renewing themselves. Even if some toxins were to fall through the cracks, your liver would simply kick in and dismantle them. After that, your kidneys take over, flushing them straight out of your body, so nothing hangs around for very long.

➤ **BOTTOM LINE:** A clean diet that's filled with naturally antioxidant- and phytonutrient-rich produce, beans, and whole grains can give you all the cancer-thwarting nutrients you need.

➤ **FACT** A 2012 study found that eating cruciferous vegetables at least once a week reduced a person's risk of esophageal, throat, colon, breast, and kidney cancers up to 32 percent.

➤ **SMART TIP** Heat deactivates the enzyme that converts glucosinolates into isothiocyanates, so cook cruciferous vegetables as little as possible. Better yet, serve them raw to preserve more of their cancer-fighting power and chop them into small pieces to release the most glucosinolates possible.

Where to Find Them:
ARUGULA

This leafy green might look like spinach, but it's actually a cruciferous vegetable like broccoli and Brussels sprouts. Just like the rest of its cruciferous relatives, it's rich in isothiocyanates, especially one named erucin. Erucin may halt the growth and proliferation of breast cancer cells. If that weren't enough, erucin is a natural detoxifier, activating enzymes that dismantle carcinogens. Right now, researchers aren't 100 percent sure how erucin works, but they suspect that it tells cells when it's time to die.

➤ **GOOD TO KNOW!** Two more vegetables are high in erucin: Chinese cabbage and kohlrabi, which is part of the turnip family.

➤ **QUICK IDEAS** For a new spin on pasta primavera, toss fresh arugula with whole-wheat pasta, garlic, olive oil, and halved grape tomatoes. Or, try it in a salad with cannellini beans, olive oil, lemon juice, and a little Parmesan.

➤ **DID YOU KNOW?** Only 5 calories per cup, arugula is one of the most slimming foods on the planet.

➤ **BONUS!** Arugula is an easy way to get more bone-friendly vitamin K. One cup packs in a quarter of your day's worth.

RECIPES
- Mediterranean Shrimp and Bulgur, page 184
- Tuna Fennel Wrap, page 156

CAULIFLOWER

Milder in flavor than broccoli, cauliflower doesn't get nearly the love of its cruciferous cousin, despite the fact that it contains practically as many glucosinolates. And its meaty texture makes it an ideal way to cut calories and saturated fat from the likes of red meat. (To find out more about the cancer-fighting perks of limiting beef and more, check out "Downsize It! Red Meat" on page 56.)

➤ QUICK IDEA Toss microwaved cauliflower with your favorite vinaigrette for a speedy side dish. How to prepare: Cut one cauliflower head into florets, place in a microwave-safe dish, and cover with an inch of water. Then cover and microwave for 5–7 minutes.

➤ SMART TIP Cauliflower can make a lighter mashed potato. Just boil, mash, and swap it in for half the potatoes you'd normally use.

➤ BONUS! One cup of cooked cauliflower gives you 73 percent of your day's worth of vitamin C.

➤ GOOD TO KNOW! Collard greens, mustard greens, bok choy, rutabaga, horseradish, and wasabi are glucosinolate powerhouses as well.

RECIPES
◆ Cauliflower Curry Stew, page 166
◆ Cauliflower Mac 'n' Cheese, page 168

PLANT PROTEIN

What It Is: Protein isn't only in meat, poultry, fish, eggs, and dairy. You can also find it in plant foods like beans, lentils, edamame, tofu, nuts, seeds, and whole grains. Yet, there's one major difference: animal foods provide complete protein—protein that supplies all the amino acids your body needs but can't make itself (see "What Are Amino Acids?" below). Plants usually do not, though there is a small handful of exceptions: soy, quinoa, and chia seeds.

How It Fights Cancer: People who favor plant protein also tend to eat less protein overall than carnivores. That might sound like a drawback, but cancer-wise a little less protein may be an advantage. A recent study looked at the impact of differing amounts

WHAT ARE AMINO ACIDS?

Your body can't absorb protein whole, so after you eat foods containing protein, your digestive system breaks it down into smaller components known as amino acids. Your body then uses these protein building blocks to construct muscle, enzymes, hormones, and antibodies.

Since most plants don't contain all of the amino acids your body needs, people often assume they're inferior. That's a shame, because eating different kinds of plant foods—whole grains, beans, nuts, and seeds—can supply all of the amino acids you require to stay strong and healthy. Even better, plant protein usually travels with other good-for-you nutrients such as phytonutrients, antioxidants, and fiber *and* contains absolutely zero cholesterol and very little saturated fat.

Red meat

If you love a juicy steak, you don't need to swear off red meat completely—but you might want to eat less of it. Unlike heart disease, it's not so much the saturated fat in red meat that's the problem. Red meat, including beef, lamb, and certain cuts of pork, contains a special kind of iron known as heme iron. Never heard of it? Iron in food is found in two different forms. There's heme iron from animal foods like meat, poultry and fish, and non-heme iron in plants such as grains, beans, and vegetables. While heme iron is much easier to absorb than its non-heme sibling, it has one downside: too much of it can encourage the formation of cancer-causing free radicals that attack the cells that line your colon.

Still, it's safe to eat up to 18 ounces of red meat per week, according to the American Institute of Cancer Research. That's the equivalent of roughly four small steaks, each about the size of your palm or a deck of cards. If you can manage to eat less, you'll reap even more benefits. A recent *Archives of Internal Medicine* study found that swapping in one daily serving of fish, poultry, nuts, beans, lowfat dairy, or whole grains for red meat can cut your risk of dying an early death from any cause by up to 19 percent. The meal plan in this chapter gives you a lot of great options!

of protein in the diets of people between the ages of 50 and 65. Those who downed more than 20 percent of their calories from protein were 75 percent more likely to die an early death and four times more likely to die of cancer than those who consumed half as much protein. Why is too much protein a problem when it comes to cancer? Protein causes your body to make a hormone that's related to insulin known as insulin-like growth factor, or IGF-1. And just like excess insulin isn't good for your blood sugar, too much IGF-1 spells trouble in a different way: speeding up cell division and increasing cancer-causing DNA damage.

➤ FACT Making your diet up to 20 percent plant protein may potentially deactivate carcinogens.

➤ SMART TIP Going meatless even one day a week can be a healthy move. Flip to the "Nutritionist's Note" on page 60 to learn how.

Where to Find It:
BLACK BEANS
By age 50, roughly 25 percent of Americans will have colon polyps, those troublesome little precursors to colon cancer. By age 70, that number doubles. Luckily, beans can help. Eating beans four times a week can cut your polyp risk by a third. How? After you digest beans, they produce a special fatty acid known as butyrate that nourishes colon cells so they stay healthy and cancer-free. Even though all beans are beneficial, black beans may be an especially good pick. When researchers fed rodents either their usual diet or one that was loaded with black beans, the black bean eaters

GRILL SAFER

For those times when you do eat meat, the way you cook it can make a big difference. Grilling or cooking any kind of meat (chicken and fish included) at searing hot temperatures leads to the formation of cancer-causing substances called heterocyclic amines (HCAs) and polycyclic aromatic hydrocarbons (PAHs). If you're going to throw a piece of steak, chicken, or fish on the barbecue, try to cook it at as low a temperature as possible and trim it of all visible fat to keep the flame from flaring up. Marinating your meat for at least 30 minutes beforehand also helps, thanks to acid-containing ingredients like vinegar that hinder PAH formation.

developed nearly 60 percent fewer colon cancers than those who enjoyed their usual chow.

➤ **FACT** Beans can also reduce your odds of developing oral, esophageal, stomach, and kidney cancers.

➤ **SMART TIP** Swap in black beans for half the meat you'd usually use in tacos or sloppy joes.

➤ **DID YOU KNOW?** Beans are natural appetite suppressants, helping you stay lean and trim, thanks to 15 grams each of protein and fiber in just 1 cup.

➤ **BONUS!** Black beans are an easy way to rack up folate, another nutrient that combats cancer. One cup gives you 40 percent of your daily fill.

RECIPES
- Black Bean Burger Salad, page 149
- Black Bean Tomato Soup, page 150
- Breakfast Burrito, page 138
- Huevos Rancheros, page 140

PEANUT BUTTER

What a woman eats as a tween or teen may have a profound impact on her breast health years later. When researchers at several leading universities tracked the diets of more than 9,000 women, they found that those who ate peanuts or peanut butter at least twice a week between the ages of 9 and 15 were 39 percent less likely to develop benign breast disease, or BBD, as adults. (Benign breast disease itself isn't cancerous, but it can raise a woman's chances of developing breast cancer.) Why are peanuts so helpful at such an early age? Adolescence is when breast tissue forms rapidly, so eating protective nutrients found in peanuts, such as vegetable protein, fiber, phytosterols, and folate, ensures that it develops properly, guarding against cancers later on. That said, eating them helps at *any* age.

➤ **SMART TIP** If you're allergic to peanut butter, sunflower, almond, and soy nut butter are all tasty, protein-packed substitutes. Swap them in for peanut butter in any of the recipes in this book.

➤ **QUICK IDEA** Use nut butter instead of cream cheese or butter on your toast, English muffin, or bagel at breakfast.

➤ **DID YOU KNOW?** Reduced-fat peanut butter can actually contain more calories than the traditional kind due to added sugars.

THE TRUTH ABOUT
Processed meat

While you don't have to ditch red meat entirely, processed meat is another story. Just 3.5 ounces a day can boost your colon cancer risk by 36 percent. That's why the American Institute for Cancer Research recommends steering clear of these foods, except for the very occasional treat. Processed meat isn't just meat that's preserved with chemicals. It's anything that's been salted, cured, or smoked. That even includes healthy-sounding picks like sliced deli turkey, nitrite-free bacon, or smoked chicken, as well as the usual suspects like hot dogs, sausage, salami, pepperoni, and ham. How can that be? Just like grilling, smoking generates dangerous PAHs. And heavy salting has been linked to an increased risk of stomach cancer, not to mention higher blood pressure.

➤ BOTTOM LINE: Instead of eating processed meats for lunch, reach for canned tuna or salmon, hard-cooked eggs, nut butters, hummus, or roasted chicken. They all deliver the protein you need to keep going all afternoon without the downsides of processed meats.

➤ GOOD TO KNOW! Ever considered buying peanut butter that's been fortified with omega-3 fats? Save your money. The amount of added omega-3s is so small, it's not worth the added cost.

➤ BONUS! Two tablespoons of peanut butter deliver nearly 20 percent of your daily vitamin E, a nutrient needed to keep your immune system strong and your skin healthy.

RECIPES
- PB & Banana Oatmeal, page 142
- PB & Banana "Sandwich," page 225
- Soba Noodles with Shrimp, Snow Peas, Carrots, and Edamame, page 200

QUINOA
Beans, nuts, peas, and lentils aren't the only way to load up on plant protein. With 8 grams of protein per cooked cup, this ancient grain supplies as much protein as a glass of milk. And, as you may remember, quinoa contains *complete* protein, like the kind you'd get from meat, chicken, or fish. Ready in just 15 minutes flat, it could be the fastest-cooking whole grain around! Just be sure to rinse quinoa before cooking, to remove any bitter-tasting residue.

➤ QUICK IDEA Try quinoa for breakfast with chopped dried tart cherries, cinnamon, and walnuts; as a swap for couscous in a side salad; or as a filling for stuffed tomatoes or peppers.

➤ SMART TIP Cook up a big pot of quinoa. Then, divide it into single-serve portions in plastic bags and pop them in the freezer so you'll always have healthy whole grains on hand.

➤ GOOD TO KNOW! Quinoa is packed with fiber, boasting 5 grams per cooked cup. Because it soaks up lots of water, it's super-filling and curbs your appetite.

MARINATE IT!

MARINADE	BEST FOR	MAKE IT
Ginger-Teriyaki	Tofu or Shrimp	1/3 cup reduced sodium soy sauce + 2 sliced scallions + 2 tablespoons chopped ginger + 2 tablespoons brown sugar
Red Wine-Rosemary	Steak	1/4 cup dry red wine + 1 clove chopped garlic + 1 tablespoon each: tomato paste, Dijon-style mustard, balsamic vinegar, and chopped fresh rosemary
Basil-Orange	Chicken	1 1/2 teaspoons each orange and lemon zest + 4 tablespoons orange juice + 1/3 cup lemon juice + 1 tablespoon olive oil + 1/2 cup chopped basil leaves

➤ **BONUS!** Quinoa is rich in zinc and iron, minerals that help your skin and nails look their best.

RECIPES
- Orange and Apricot Quinoa, page 141
- Quinoa Cannellini Salad, page 154

OTHER CANCER-FIGHTING POWER FOODS
BUTTERNUT SQUASH
How It Keeps Cancer At Bay: It's rich in alpha- and beta-carotene and beta-crypto-xanthin.

You've heard of beta-carotene? Well, say hello to its friends alpha-carotene and beta-cryptoxanthin. These plant pigments belong to a family of compounds known as carotenoids that may ward off kidney cancer. When researchers looked at the diets of nearly three-quarters of a million people, they found that those who consumed the most of these three nutrients were up to 18 percent less likely to develop kidney cancer, thanks to their ability to keep cell growth in check.

➤ **GOOD TO KNOW!** Carrots, pumpkin, and sweet potatoes are also packed with carotenoids.

➤ **DID YOU KNOW?** With 80 calories per cup, butternut squash contains less than half the calories you'd get from sweet potatoes.

➤ **SMART TIP** Many supermarkets carry fresh, precut, peeled butternut squash in the produce section—no peeling or chopping necessary!

➤ **QUICK IDEA** For a satisfying side dish, toss cubed butternut squash with olive oil, cinnamon, sea salt, and black pepper, and roast in a 400°F oven for 30 minutes.

➤ **BONUS!** A cup of cooked butternut squash gives you 41 percent of your daily vitamin C.

GINGER

How It Keeps Cancer At Bay: It's rich in compounds that fight ovarian cancer.

Health experts don't know specifically what causes ovarian cancer, but they suspect a protein called nuclear factor of kappaB (or NF-κB, for short) is involved. Left unchecked, NF-κB can change the genetic blueprint of your DNA, causing cells to grow out of control. Eating more ginger could help. According to research from the University of Michigan, ginger contains special compounds, such as 6-shogaol and gingerol, which stop NF-κB in its tracks.

➤ **QUICK IDEA** Blend 1 teaspoon of fresh ginger into a smoothie with some frozen strawberries and orange juice.

➤ **SMART TIP** When buying fresh ginger, look for pieces with smooth skin. Wrap it in plastic, and it will stay fresh in your fridge for 3 weeks.

➤ **BONUS!** Ginger can relieve nausea, menstrual cramps, and arthritis pain.

- Spiced Pork Tenderloins with Mango Salsa, page 202

LENTILS

How They Keep Cancer At Bay: They're rich in folate.

Lentils are bursting with the B vitamin folate, a nutrient that's critical for maintaining healthy DNA. Think it's easier to pop a multivitamin or folic acid supplement instead? Keep in mind that folate and folic acid (which you get from supplements) are not the same nutrient, though they are closely related.

Folic acid is the man-made form of folate. While you can't get too much folate from foods, you can definitely get too much folic acid from supplements. And this may actually encourage cancer growth — particularly if a tumor has already formed, since folate helps cells reproduce normally and excessive amounts of folate can speed up the process. For maximum protection, get your folate from foods and skip the supplements.

➤ **QUICK IDEA** Toss ½ cup of cooked lentils into your salad or soup, and you'll rack up nearly half your day's worth of folate (women need 400 micrograms a day).

➤ **GOOD TO KNOW!** Spinach, asparagus, oranges, lima beans, and chickpeas are all full of natural folate.

➤ **BONUS!** Lentils are jammed with potassium for better blood pressure. One cup delivers 731 milligrams. That's more than you'd get from two small bananas!

RECIPES
- Slow Cooker Italian Lentil and Vegetable Stew, page 199

PUMPKIN

How It Keeps Cancer At Bay: It's rich in cucurmosin.

Despite a decline in overall cancer rates, pancreatic cancer is on the rise. While there are many pancreatic cancer risk factors you can't control, there are some that are within your power, such as avoiding tobacco and maintaining a healthy body weight, especially since being obese ups your pancreatic cancer risk by 20 percent. And add pumpkin to your meal rotation. It's a top source of cucurmosin, a plant compound that prevents pancreatic cancer by curbing uncontrolled cell growth.

➤ **SMART TIP** Keep a couple of cans of puréed pumpkin on hand to spoon into oatmeal, whole-wheat pancakes, or smoothies.

HOW TO BEAT BEAN BLOAT

If beans make you gassy and bloated, start by adding them to your diet slowly, say once or twice a week. That will give your digestive system a chance to adjust to their unique carbohydrates, which can be difficult to digest if you're not used to eating them. Rinsing canned beans can wash some of these carbs away and make them easier on your stomach, too.

➤ **QUICK IDEA** Explore pumpkin's savory side by stirring it into macaroni and cheese, risotto, polenta, or even grits.

➤ **GOOD TO KNOW!** With only 84 calories and 7 grams of satisfying fiber per cup, pumpkin can help keep off unwanted weight.

➤ **BONUS!** Pumpkin is one of the very best sources of vitamin A, a nutrient needed for healthy skin and a strong immune system. One cup gives you nearly three times your daily fill of this vitamin.

RECIPE

- Cumin-Spiced Pumpkin Soup, page 217
- Pumpkin Smoothie, page 225
- Healthy Pumpkin Bread, page 222

TROUT

How It Keeps Cancer At Bay: It's rich in vitamin D.

Fatty fish, like trout, is one of the few foods that provide meaningful amounts of protective vitamin D—just one palm-sized serving of trout supplies more than your entire day's worth. For some time, experts have observed that people with higher levels of vitamin D in their blood tend to have less cancer. The answer may lie with vitamin D's ability to slow down cell division, ensuring that cells reproduce in an orderly fashion. In addition, vitamin D regulates cells' ability to specialize, or carry out the jobs for which they were uniquely intended. That's important because cancer cells don't specialize—they just grow and grow and grow.

➤ **GOOD TO KNOW!** You can also find vitamin D in salmon and sardines.

➤ **FACT** Up until age 70, women require at least 600 international units (IU) of vitamin

---

YOU ASKED
Does beta-carotene cause lung cancer?

No, provided it's in its natural form.
Carotenoids, particularly alpha-carotene and beta-cryptoxanthin, have been found to protect against lung cancer, but only when they come from food, not supplements. In fact, a small handful of studies have linked beta-carotene supplements to *increased* lung cancer risk among people who smoke, although experts aren't sure exactly why. To be on the safe side, get your carotenoids from food, not pills.

D a day (IU is measurement used for certain vitamins such as A, D, and E). Women over the age of 70 need a minimum of 800 IU. You can learn even more about how much vitamin D you need and how to get it on page 93 of chapter 6.

➤ **QUICK IDEA** Broiling is one of the fastest ways to cook trout. Just brush with olive oil, season with fresh or dried herbs (try parsley or chives), and broil, skin-side down, for five minutes.

➤ **SMART TIP** Some lake trout populations are dwindling due to overfishing. For a more sustainable choice, the Monterey Bay Aquarium's Seafood Watch recommends farmed rainbow trout instead.

➤ **BONUS!** Trout is an impressive source of vitamin B$_{12}$, which keeps your brain sharp and your nervous system healthy. One 4-ounce serving gives you twice your daily dose.

CHECKLIST
For cancer-prevention

❍ Working more fiber into your diet can help reduce your risk of cancer, plus it keeps you full and promotes digestive health. To get your 25 daily grams, include fiber-rich fruits, vegetables, beans, and whole grains at every meal and most snacks.

❍ Vegetables are one of the most important foods for cancer prevention. To make sure you get enough, think convenience. Frozen peas, prewashed and bagged arugula, and precut butternut squash make it simple.

❍ Salads are an easy way to load up on produce. Make yours even healthier by tossing in cruciferous greens like arugula or kale.

❍ For mornings when you hardly have time to eat breakfast, keep a couple of boxes of whole-grain cereal on hand.

❍ Load up on speedy sources of cancer-fighting plant protein such as peanut butter, quinoa, and canned lentils and black beans.

❍ Choose natural sources of folate, such as spinach, asparagus, oranges, peanuts, and beans, and steer clear of folic acid supplements.

❍ Try going meatless at least one day a week.

❍ Next time you eat fish, try trout, salmon, or sardines for a vitamin D boost plus healthy fats.

❍ If you drink, limit alcohol to no more than one drink a day. In terms of serving sizes, that's a 5-ounce glass of wine, a 12-ounce beer, or 1.5 ounces of vodka, gin, or whiskey.

One-week cancer-fighting meal plan

	BREAKFAST	LUNCH	DINNER
DAY 1	PB & Banana Oatmeal*	Veggie Burger Parmesan* 1 cup arugula drizzled with 1 tablespoon balsamic vinaigrette	4 ounces broiled or grilled trout ½ cup brown rice, prepared according to package directions 1 cup cauliflower florets sautéed in 2 teaspoons olive oil
DAY 2	Better-for-You Blueberry Waffles*	Brown Rice Edamame Salad*	Slow Cooker Italian Lentil and Vegetable Stew* ½ cup sliced strawberries mixed with ½ cup pomegranate seeds
DAY 3	Breakfast Burrito*	Grilled Shrimp Caesar* 12 whole-wheat pita chips	Orange-Soy Tofu Stir-Fry* ⅓ cup quinoa, prepared according to package directions
DAY 4	Pomegranate-Apricot Breakfast Crostini*	Tuna Fennel Wrap*	Cauliflower Mac 'n' Cheese* 1 medium tomato, sliced and drizzled with 1 teaspoon balsamic vinegar
DAY 5	1 cup spoon-sized shredded wheat with ½ cup sliced strawberries and 1 cup 1% milk	Spread 2 tablespoons nut butter and 1 tablespoon strawberry jam on an 8-inch whole-wheat pita. Top with ½ sliced banana. Fold into wrap.	Grilled Chicken Salad with Avocado and Grapefruit* ½ cup no-salt-added, rinsed and drained canned black beans, warmed in the microwave
DAY 6	Orange and Apricot Quinoa*	Barley-Stuffed Pepper*	Cumin-Spiced Pumpkin Soup* Curried Rice with Shrimp and Peas*
DAY 7	Mash one fifth avocado and spread on 1 slice whole-wheat toast. Drizzle with Sriracha hot sauce, if desired. 1 egg scrambled in 1 teaspoon butter ½ grapefruit	Black Bean Tomato Soup*	Slow Cooker Butternut Squash Barley Risotto* 1 cup arugula, ½ cup rinsed and drained no-salt-added canned cannellini beans and 1 tablespoon balsamic vinaigrette

*Recipe included in chapter 9

Pumpkin Smoothie*
35 peanuts

¼ cup part-skim ricotta mixed with a dash of cinnamon on 8 small whole-wheat crackers
1 sliced bell pepper dipped in ¼ cup hummus

1 apple with 1 tablespoon nut butter
1 piece of reduced-fat string cheese + 1 cup grapes

8-ounce nonfat green tea latte
1 nut-based snack bar

Unlimited broccoli and cauliflower florets dipped in your favorite salsa
Chocolate Chili Popcorn*

Spicy Trail Mix*
Chia Pudding*

¾ cup edamame
Mix ¼ cup pomegranate seeds into 6 ounces lowfat vanilla yogurt

CHAPTER 5

Boost Your Brainpower

Of the five million Americans with Alzheimer's disease, nearly two thirds are female. Pick the proper Power Foods to preserve your mental clarity and frame of mind.

WHAT CAUSES MEMORY PROBLEMS AND MOOD DISORDERS

Your brain is an amazing organ made of 100 billion neurons. Its cells are in constant communication with each other, sending signals back and forth 24/7 via connections known as synapses. To work efficiently, your brain needs fuel, namely glucose. It also requires vitamins, minerals, and healthy fats. Without enough of these, the conversation between neurons can get interrupted—and you may find that you're tired and unmotivated.

Certain nutrients help your brain manufacture chemicals that cause you to drift off at night, too. If you're lacking them, sleep can become an issue, making you feel more lethargic and sluggish. Mood-wise, you may

WHO IS MOST LIKELY TO SUFFER FROM DEPRESSION?

One in 10 Americans struggles with this disease. You're more likely to be at risk if you:

- Are female
- Are between the ages of 45 and 64
- Suffer from cardiovascular disease
- Have a family history of depression
- Never completed high school
- Are black, Hispanic, or multiracial
- Are unemployed
- Don't have health insurance

start to feel sad, anxious, and stressed. The food-mood connection is so real that studies show that people who eat better are actually less likely to battle the blues and anxiety than those who have diets heavy in refined grains, fried foods, and sugar.

Well before you reach old age, healthier diets that contain lots of fruits, vegetables, whole grains, nuts, and fish yet are low in meat, poultry, refined grains, and animal fat have been linked to better overall memory. And the food you choose makes a major difference in your long-term recall and problem-solving skills. If that sounds like a big deal, it is, especially for women. By the time you reach your 60s, your chances of having memory-robbing Alzheimer's disease are one in six. And after age 65, your odds of Alzheimer's double every 5 years.

THE GOOD NEWS

A brain-friendly diet can go a long way in helping you stay mentally keen and balanced. It starts with the same foundation you'd choose for a healthy heart: lots of produce; whole grains; some good fats from vegetable oils, nuts, and fish; and limited cholesterol, saturated fats,

FOR A YOUNGER BRAIN, HAVE MORE FUN!

There's another facet to brain health that has nothing to do with what you eat or how much you move. It's having fun. While experts aren't sure exactly why, they've found that staying mentally busy with activities that challenge your mind, like playing board games, doing puzzles, reading, or playing a musical instrument, keeps you quick-witted as you get older. That same is true for staying social by spending time and maintaining close relationships with friends and family.

and trans fats. How does the heart-brain connection work? In the same way that your heart requires ample blood flow to deliver oxygen and nutrients, so does your brain.

Watching the scale helps, too, making it extra important to keep an eye on portion sizes and stay active. Excess weight has such a profound effect on brain health that being obese at midlife can double your chances of Alzheimer's disease later on (read more about "The Body Weight–Memory Link" on page 76).

SUPER NUTRIENTS AND POWER FOODS
COMPLEX CARBOHYDRATES

What They Are: Carbohydrates come in two basic forms: simple and complex. Simple carbs from foods like soda, juice, and sweets are essentially sugars (you learned about these types of carbs—called refined carbohydrates—in chapter 3). There are also simple carbs in whole fruit, but because fruit's fiber slows down the release of its sugars, it's not in the same category as other sugary simple carbs. Then, there are complex carbohydrates from potatoes, bread, cereal, pasta, and rice. These carbs come in the form of starch, which requires more time to break down to glucose, your body's preferred source of fuel. As a result, they provide a more steady sugar release that keeps your body—and brain—fueled for hours. Of these, the very best choices are whole grains (which you also read about in chapter 3), since their complex carbs take longer to break down and digest.

How They Boost Brainpower: Your brain requires an enormous amount of glucose for fuel, using an incredible 60 percent of your body's glucose when you're sitting or lying down. But where those carbs come from matters—a lot. You may remember from chapter 3 that sugar-filled foods can send your blood sugar into a tailspin, causing it to soar and then quickly plummet. Slowly digested complex carbohydrates, on the other hand, keep blood sugar nice and balanced. What does this have to do with your brain? Health experts are

THE TRUTH ABOUT
Paleo diets

On the surface, Paleo diets seem like a smart eating plan. Based on the premise that we should eat like our Paleolithic ancestors (i.e., cavemen), the Paleo diet is filled with lean meat, poultry, and seafood, fruits, vegetables, nuts, and certain oils, such as olive and coconut oils. From these, you get plenty of protein and, if you choose carefully, fiber to keep you full and steady your blood sugar. Plus, you'll never have to count calories.

Sounds pretty good, right? The trouble with Paleo diets is that for all of the foods you can eat, there are even more that you can't. All grains, beans, and legumes (including peanuts), dairy products, potatoes, and many vegetable oils are strictly off limits. That can get boring pretty quickly.

➤ **BOTTOM LINE:** *Any* diet that eliminates one or more food groups should send up an immediate red flag, as it's likely to rob you of important Power Foods and Super Nutrients that your body needs to stay strong and fight disease.

learning that too many sugary foods may make it difficult to remember small yet important details. One study found that eating just one high-glycemic-index meal impaired memory as soon as an hour or two afterward, while low-GI carbs enhance recall. (For more on the glycemic index and how it impacts your blood sugar, turn to page 33 in chapter 3.)

Sugar-filled foods also spell memory trouble in the long run by raising your odds of insulin resistance. And insulin issues have been shown to interfere with your memory as well as your ability to process information. That's because your hippocampus, the part of your brain that helps you organize, process, and remember things, requires insulin for peak performance. So, when insulin isn't working properly, your brain can't function optimally.

➤ FACT Your brain requires so many carbs that it burns through about 30 teaspoons of glucose a day. That's anywhere from 25 to 30 percent of your daily calories.

➤ DID YOU KNOW? Carbs help you produce serotonin, a brain chemical that makes you feel happy and relaxed.

➤ GOOD TO KNOW! There's no one-size-fits-all daily recommendation for carbs. Anywhere between 45 and 65 percent of your calories is ideal, providing they're mostly complex carbs from foods such as whole grains. That translates to 170–240 grams a day, if you're on the small side, or 200–290 grams, if you're taller.

Where to Find Them:
BRAN FLAKES

There are three pieces to the perfect breakfast: slowly digested protein, fiber to keep you full, and carbs for energy. And the last part of the equation is especially important. Here's why: After a nightlong fast, your body has burned through nearly all the carbs you ate at last night's dinner, which means your brain is going to be hungry for its favorite fuel, namely carbohydrates. But don't just feed it any old kind. Reach for ones that stick to your ribs with complex carbs. And what could be easier than a bowl of bran flakes, which have just the right amount of fiber, about 5 grams per ¾ cup? (For more on choosing the best breakfast cereal, flip to "Food Label Sleuth: Cereal" on page 50.) That's enough to keep you full, but not so much that it ties your stomach in a knot (check the "Nutritionist's Note" on page 48 in chapter 4 for more smart tips).

HOW CARBS KEEP YOU HAPPY

When it comes to your mental outlook, carb quality matters, especially if you're watching your weight. When researchers put dieting volunteers on either a high- or a low-GI diet, they found that the low-GI group experienced less anxiety, depression, and fatigue. That doesn't mean you have to say good-bye to cookies, cakes, and brownies forever, but getting the bulk of your carbs from slowly digested, fiber-rich whole grains and beans could spell a more upbeat you.

On finding whole grains

In chapter 3 and this chapter, you'll read about the perks of eating more whole grains. Until recently, that wasn't necessarily easy. Now, supermarket shelves are packed with wholesome whole grains, from quinoa and brown rice to whole-wheat couscous and pasta, not to mention whole-wheat bread, bagels, and English muffins. But often, my clients are stumped when they eat out. Restaurants are offering more whole grains than in years past, but you may still have to do a little extra sleuthing to find them. The easiest way? Go ethnic. If you're in the mood for Mexican, look for a restaurant where you'll find brown rice and corn tortillas (order three corn-tortilla soft tacos, and you'll gain 5 grams of satiating fiber). Want Asian? Your options are even greater. Plenty of Chinese chains offer brown rice. Some restaurants now even serve quinoa bowls. And keep in mind that experts recommend making at least *half* of your grains whole, so the occasional plate of regular pasta is okay, too.

P.S. If your family resists whenever you put whole grains on the table, try this nutritionist-approved trick: swap out half the white grains on your plate for whole grains by making a 50-50 mix of white and brown rice or regular and whole-wheat pasta.

➤ **FACT** Bran could also help you live longer. A 2010 *Circulation* study found that women who ate the most bran were 28 percent less likely to die an early death than those who ate the least.

➤ **GOOD TO KNOW!** Three-quarters of a cup of bran flakes has only 98 calories.

➤ **SMART TIP** Don't just save bran cereal for breakfast. Try it with almonds and your favorite sliced fruit for a light lunch or satisfying snack.

➤ **BONUS!** Bran flakes are often fortified with iron, with many brands supplying 45 percent or more of your daily quota. Iron is a key player for keeping red blood cells strong and vibrant so they can ferry oxygen to your brain. Without enough, you may feel tired, lethargic, and unable to concentrate. Plus, you'll be more prone to depression and PMS.

POPCORN

Usually, most crunchy snacks are made of nutritionally empty processed carbs. Not popcorn. For starters, it's a whole grain, so it's packed with complex carbohydrates. It's also amazingly low in calories (just 93 per 3 cups of air-popped popcorn), yet high in satiating fiber (nearly 4 grams for the same amount). Even more surprising, popcorn is filled with brain-supporting compounds called polyphenols (you'll learn more about these later in this chapter on page 75). Just one serving dishes up as many of these helpful compounds as two servings of fruit.

➤ **FACT** A 2008 study in the *Journal of the American Dietetic Association* found that popcorn eaters consume two and a half times more whole grains and 22 percent more fiber than people who don't munch on this snack.

➤ **GOOD TO KNOW!** All popcorn is whole grain, but air-popped is best, as it has no added fat, salt, or preservatives.

➤ **QUICK IDEA** For an instant flavor kick, sprinkle popcorn with a few shakes of cinnamon, cumin, curry, or chili powder.

➤ **QUICK IDEA** For a filling 150-calorie snack, mix 3 cups air-popped popcorn with a small handful (about 12) pistachios or peanuts.

———

RECIPE
◆ Chocolate Chili Popcorn, page 224

WHOLE-WHEAT COUSCOUS

If you've been dragging all day, the culprit could be last night's dinner, especially if it was too heavy. Fatty meals relax the valve that normally seals your stomach off from your esophagus. When that valve opens, a rush of stomach acids shoots back upward, causing a gnawing case of heartburn, which can make it hard to get a restful night's sleep. Even if heartburn isn't an issue for you, research reveals that people who eat more fat tend to slumber less and don't have as much restorative REM sleep. Lightening things up at dinnertime by eating fewer fatty foods and more whole grains like fluffy whole-wheat couscous can help. At only 175 calories per cooked cup, it has 20 percent fewer calories than a 220-calorie cup of spaghetti. Plus, it only takes 10 minutes to prepare, so it's an especially quick way to work in more whole grains.

➤ **QUICK IDEA** Couscous pairs perfectly with beans. For a Mexican spin, try it with black beans, corn, scallions, and minced jalapeño.

Or think Mediterranean by pairing it with chickpeas, tomatoes, basil, Kalamata olives, and a sprinkle of feta cheese.

➤ **DID YOU KNOW?** The complex carbs in whole-wheat couscous help you produce more calming serotonin. In addition to helping you relax, serotonin helps your body make melatonin, a key player for a better night's sleep. So eat up, and drift off faster.

———

RECIPES
◆ Couscous with Chickpeas, page 151
◆ Greek-Style Tilapia, page 175

WHOLE-WHEAT TORTILLAS

Next time you need whole grains on the go, reach for a whole-wheat tortilla. Unlike cooked grains like barley, oatmeal, bulgur, brown rice, quinoa, and couscous, tortillas don't require a fork or spoon. Plus, they give you all the whole-grain goodness of whole-wheat bread. Even better, they boast an incredibly low glycemic index of 30, compared to whole-wheat bread's 71, for more slowly released energy.

➤ **SMART TIP** Some tortillas are as big as 12 inches wide, with upwards of 300 calories. Look for tortillas that are about 8 inches across and less than 150 calories. And scour the ingredient list to be sure the whole-wheat flour is the very first ingredient.

➤ **DID YOU KNOW?** Corn tortillas are also made with whole grains, so they're a good pick, too.

———

RECIPES
◆ Breakfast Burrito, page 138
◆ Tuna Fennel Wrap, page 156

may become depressed, confused, anemic, and more prone to heart disease.

How It Boosts Brainpower: Mood-wise, vitamin B_6 helps convert the amino acid tryptophan into the feel-good brain chemical serotonin—low levels of B_6 can make you feel anxious and depressed. (To learn more about how amino acids work, turn to page 89 in chapter 4.)

B_6 may also keep your brain younger. Along with its B vitamin siblings, B_{12} and folate, vitamin B_6 lowers amounts of the amino acid homocysteine in your blood. That's a plus because high homocysteine levels have been linked to cognitive decline and Alzheimer's disease as well as heart disease. According to a recent British study, these nutrients can actually reduce homocysteine-related brain shrinkage associated with Alzheimer's.

➤ **BONUS!** A small number of studies have found that B_6 is helpful for managing monthly PMS-related moodiness.

➤ **GOOD TO KNOW!** As you get older, your B_6 needs to increase. You require 1.3 milligrams a day up until age 50, and 1.5 milligrams afterward.

VITAMIN B_6

What It Is: This B vitamin helps you make oxygen-carrying red blood cells, keeps your metabolism working properly, and builds a strong immune system. Because vitamin B_6 is so important for your immune system, it should also be on your radar if you have an autoimmune disease such as celiac disease, rheumatoid arthritis, ulcerative colitis, or Crohn's disease. Without enough B_6, you

Where to Find It:
BAKED POTATOES

Potatoes are nutrition stars *and* good-mood food. Loaded with complex carbs and vitamin B_6 (one medium baked potato gives you 40 percent of your day's worth), these tubers boost serotonin levels. Why bake your potatoes instead of boiling them? Boiling causes nearly a quarter of a potato's potassium and vitamin B_6 to leach out into the cooking water.

➤ **BONUS!** Potatoes boast more than 60 different kinds of phytochemicals and nearly as many polyphenols as Brussels sprouts, broccoli, and spinach.

➤ **DID YOU KNOW?** Baked potatoes are lower in calories than you might expect. One medium potato contains only 161 calories.

➤ **SMART TIP** Eat potatoes with the skin on, and you'll rack up 50 percent more fiber and a third more potassium than if you take the skin off.

———

RECIPE
◆ Baked Potato "Burrito Bowl," page 148

BANANAS
Next time you're having a rough afternoon, grab a banana. They're a top source of soothing complex carbs. Plus, one medium banana delivers a third of your day's mood-enhancing B_6. If you're headed to the gym, they can also help you power through your sweat session. Researchers at Appalachian State University found that bananas were as effective for fueling cyclists' workouts as a sports drink.

➤ **GOOD TO KNOW!** With 3 grams of filling fiber, a medium banana is practically guaranteed to help you stay full and focused all afternoon—for just 104 calories.

➤ **BONUS!** Bananas offer up more potassium than practically any other fruit. One banana gives you 422 milligrams worth, or 9 percent of your daily dose.

———

RECIPES
◆ Creamy Orange Banana Waffle, page 139
◆ PB & Banana Oatmeal, page 142
◆ PB & Banana "Sandwich," page 225
◆ Pumpkin Smoothie, page 225
◆ Sunrise Smoothie, page 144
◆ Tropical Greek Yogurt Breakfast Parfait, page 145

FIVE QUICK IDEAS FOR OVERRIPE BANANAS

1 Slice and freeze them, so you'll always have some on hand to toss into smoothies.

2 Whip up a batch of banana muffins or banana bread.

3 Dice and fold them into whole-wheat pancakes.

4 Purée them and mix into Greek yogurt with a pinch of nutmeg.

5 Put them in the refrigerator. They'll turn brown, but they're still fine to eat.

VITAMIN B_{12}
What It Is: This B vitamin keeps your nervous system and red blood cells healthy. Without enough, you'll feel tired, weak, and generally run down. You may also feel depressed and develop a major case of brain fog—that frustrating feeling when you can't seem to concentrate no matter how hard you try.

How It Boosts Brainpower: Even though most young adults get enough B_{12}, this nutrient becomes more of a concern after you turn 50. In fact, up to 30 percent of people over age 50 don't absorb enough of this vitamin. Why? At that age, your stomach starts to produce less acid. That may sound like a good thing (especially if you've been wrestling with heartburn), but B$_{12}$ in food doesn't travel alone. Instead, it's tightly attached to protein. And stomach acid is what uncouples them. If you're over age 50, consider a senior formula multivitamin, in addition to trying to eat more foods with B$_{12}$.

➤ **FACT** You're more likely to be B$_{12}$-deficient if you have celiac or Crohn's disease or if you've had stomach surgery. Turn to "You Asked" on page 75 to learn more about the link between celiac disease and brain health.

➤ **GOOD TO KNOW!** Top sources of B$_{12}$ include trout, salmon, tuna, lean beef, and fortified cereal. Eating a bowl of fortified bran flakes with milk, a tuna fish sandwich, and a container of lowfat yogurt provides your entire day's worth (2.4 micrograms).

➤ **SMART TIP** Antacids can interfere with vitamin B$_{12}$ absorption. If you take these for heartburn, speak to your doctor about a supplement.

Where to Find It:
SHRIMP

When it comes to brain health, vitamin B$_{12}$ is one nutrient you don't want to skimp on. In addition to keeping red blood cells healthy, manufacturing neurotransmitters, and lowering homocysteine, an amino acid that can

harm your heart, this vitamin helps maintain the myelin sheath, the membrane that surrounds the nerves in your brain and spinal cord. Concerned you're not getting enough B$_{12}$? Consider seafood. A 3-ounce serving of shrimp (about 12 large shrimp) gives you 39 percent of your daily dose. Since shrimp freezes beautifully, it's easy to keep on hand. And because you can thaw it under cold running water, you don't have to defrost it in your fridge overnight—making it ideal for spur-of-the-moment meals.

➤ **QUICK IDEA** For a B$_{12}$-packed update on pasta marinara, try pasta fra diavolo. To make it, sauté shrimp with garlic, crushed red pepper flakes, and olive oil. Then toss with cooked pasta and your favorite marinara sauce.

➤ **GOOD TO KNOW!** Shrimp contains the antioxidant astaxanthin, which protects delicate brain cells from free radical strikes that age them prematurely.

➤ **SMART TIP** When it comes to the most sustainable shrimp, the Monterey Bay Aquarium's Seafood Watch recommends both wild and farmed catches from the United States. The only exception is shrimp from the Gulf of Mexico (excluding Florida), as shrimp fisheries in this region often catch sea turtles and

For some people. If you're perfectly healthy, it's unlikely that gluten is making it difficult for you to concentrate. However, people with celiac disease or a similar condition known as gluten sensitivity really do have less brain fog on a gluten-free diet. Celiac disease, which strikes 1 in every 130 people, is an autoimmune disease in which gluten, a protein in certain grains like wheat, barley, and rye, causes your body to produce antibodies that attack your small intestine. That can lead to cramps, diarrhea, poor nutrient absorption, and weight loss. It can also make you tired, irritable, and unable to focus. Unlike celiac disease, gluten sensitivity, which has been estimated to strike up to 6 percent of people, isn't an autoimmune disease, so it doesn't harm your digestive system. However, it still produces many of the same symptoms.

If you suspect you have celiac or gluten sensitivity, don't self-diagnose. Gluten-free diets cut out a *lot* of foods, which can lead to vitamin deficiencies that could make you even fuzzier than you felt to begin with. Instead, see your doctor about testing for celiac disease. Right now, there's no reliable testing for gluten sensitivity, so your doctor will want to rule out celiac first and then other mind-clouding conditions like hypothyroidism or Lyme disease. If the final results point to celiac or gluten sensitivity, then it's time to give a gluten-free diet a try. The gluten-free meal plan on page 230 in chapter 9 can show you how.

other marine species along with their shrimp. ➤ BONUS! Twelve large shrimp provide one-third of your day's phosphorus, a mineral that helps bones and teeth stay strong.

RECIPES
- Garlic Shrimp and Swiss Chard on Polenta, page 176
- Grilled Shrimp Caesar, page 152
- Curried Rice with Shrimp and Peas, page 171
- Lemon Shrimp, page 181
- Mediterranean Shrimp and Bulgur, page 184
- Soba Noodles with Shrimp, Snow Peas, Carrots, and Edamame, page 200

OTHER BRAINPOWER-BOOSTING POWER FOODS
BERRIES
How They Boost Brainpower: They're rich in polyphenols.

Your brain cells are like good friends. Normally, they talk all the time. But as they get older, and life gets in the way, they're less likely to communicate and pass along vital information. Compounds in berries called polyphenols can open up the lines of communication. How? A protective membrane surrounds every cell in your brain. When you're young, these membranes are flexible and pliable. But as you age, they gradually become tough and rigid, making it difficult for them to move freely, causing signals to travel more slowly from one cell to the next. While researchers aren't sure exactly how, they believe that polyphenols help restore that flexibility.

Berry compounds, including polyphenols, may also cushion against dementia. Even though you can't see or feel it, your brain produces an Alzheimer's-causing protein known as tau. When you're young, your brain simply dismantles tau and recycles it into proteins that it can use. However, as you age, this process becomes less efficient and tau begins to accumulate. If enough builds up, it can lead to Alzheimer's disease. Experts believe compounds in berries can jump-start your brain's protein recycling system, making tau buildup less likely.

➤ **GOOD TO KNOW!** Substances in blueberries may help you grow new neurons in your hippocampus, the part of your brain that's responsible for learning and memory.

➤ **SMART TIP** Berries become moldy quickly when they're wet, so rinse yours only right before you eat them.

➤ **QUICK IDEA** Instead of syrup on your pancakes, waffles, or French toast, make this decadent sauce from frozen berries: Toss 1 teaspoon of sugar with ½ cup frozen berries (any kind) and microwave for 1 minute, or until warm and gooey.

➤ **BONUS!** Berries are filled with fiber. Raspberries and blackberries serve up the most, with a generous 8 grams per cup.

RECIPES

THE BODY WEIGHT–MEMORY LINK

Just as weighing too much can cause insulin resistance, it can also encourage leptin resistance. Leptin is a hunger hormone that tells your brain if you're storing enough fat. Alzheimer's experts believe it may also help dismantle dementia-causing tau. How are the two related? Normally, when you have plenty of leptin, your brain thinks you've got all the padding you need to survive food scarcity—so you don't feel particularly hungry. However, when you gain too much body fat, your leptin stops functioning properly and mistakenly sends signals to your brain, telling you to eat up even though you already have plenty of cushioning. The result? You eat more, causing more weight gain and eventually memory-robbing leptin resistance, which can lead to dementia.

- Peach Blueberry Smoothie, page 142
- Roast Pork Tenderloin with Blackberry Sauce, page 193

BLACK PEPPER

How It Boosts Brainpower: It's rich in piperine.

This spice could make you thinner, thanks to its piperine, a compound that's been shown to help burn off belly fat. If you're wondering what a trimmer tummy has to do with brain health, consider this: the more you weigh, the greater your likelihood of developing Alzheimer's or dementia. When researchers compared the MRIs of middle-aged volunteers, they found that those who weighed the most had the smallest brains. An even stronger predictor of brain atrophy was visceral fat, that stubborn fat deep inside your belly that surrounds your abdominal organs. While researchers aren't sure exactly why more belly fat translates to less brain tissue, they suspect that several different mechanisms may come into play, such as increased inflammation throughout your body and brain as well as insulin resistance. True, simply sprinkling extra pepper on your food won't melt off unwanted weight, but consider it a calorie-free way to pump up the flavor in your food. Plus, pepper is a smart alternative to blood-pressure-raising salt.

➤ **FACT** When researchers at the University of Colorado served women a lunch of full-fat foods, lowfat foods, or lowfat foods with added spices, the volunteers rated the lowfat foods with the spices to be as tasty as many of the full-fat foods.

➤ **GOOD TO KNOW!** Chili powder is another spice that may help you stay slim. It contains capsaicin, a compound that dulls appetite.

➤ **BONUS!** Piperine may also protect against breast cancer.

RECIPE
- Pepper-Crusted Tuna with Sesame Asparagus, page 192

KEFIR

How It Boosts Brainpower: It's rich in probiotics.

Your digestive tract is the only system in your body that has its very own nervous system, sending signals back and forth to your brain all day long. It also produces many of the same mood-regulating neurotransmitters that your brain does, including an impressive 95 percent of your body's serotonin. That's why scientists call this tract your second brain. But serotonin doesn't just magically appear in your digestive system. Beneficial bacteria that live there make it. That's why an emerging body of research reveals that good gut bacteria, known as probiotics, can help fight anxiety and depression.

To get more of those healthy bacteria, check out kefir, a fermented milk drink with the same tangy taste of plain yogurt. This beverage contains as many as 12 different kinds of probiotic strains, more than twice as many as your average yogurt. Plus, it's cultured up to eight times as long, so the helpful bugs have more time to grow and multiply.

➤ **QUICK IDEA** Try kefir instead of yogurt in your morning or afternoon smoothie.

➤ **SMART TIP** If you like things tangy, drink kefir straight up. Just be sure to stick with the

Afternoon munchies

Step away from the vending machine. These five tricks can help you reverse your late-day energy crisis.

1 **Fortify.** Remember the last time you tried to go from lunch until dinner without some kind of snack? It can make your blood sugar plummet, causing your concentration to suffer. For maximum afternoon focus, pack a snack from home that contains a combo of complex carbs for energy plus some protein or fiber to keep you full. Top picks include a small handful of nuts plus a piece of fruit, nonfat yogurt with berries, or lowfat cheese and an apple.

2 **Up the fun factor.** If you've already gone the snack route, and you're still daydreaming about dinner, hunger might not be your issue. Perhaps you've been sitting at your desk or doing household chores for so long that you're bored silly. Shake up your afternoon with a 5-minute rope-jumping session or sneak outside for a 5- or 10-minute walk to get your blood pumping. Can't leave the building? Walk up and down the nearest stairwell.

3 **Drink up.** Even a little bit of dehydration can drain your energy. But if you're one of those people who finds water to be bland and tasteless, plain H_2O may not sound all that enticing. For flavor-filled hydration that's guaranteed to perk you up, add some mint leaves and cucumber slices to your water bottle.

4 **Take a deep breath.** When a rough day makes you want to tear into a bag of candy, take a few minutes to tune out by plugging in your earbuds, turning on some soothing music, and taking nice slow breaths.

5 **Caffeinate.** A little caffeine can go a long way toward restoring your energy and focus. But the operative word is little. Bypass the grande coffee and grab a small latte (no more than 12 ounces). You'll get just enough caffeine to power through the afternoon, plus its milk will provide some satisfying protein.

plain, unsweetened kind—it has 40 percent less sugar.

➤ GOOD TO KNOW! People who are lactose intolerant can often drink kefir without any problem, as kefir contains enzymes that make lactose easier to digest.

➤ BONUS! One 8-ounce cup of kefir has all the calcium of a glass of milk, plus a third more protein.

RECIPE
◆ Peach Blueberry Smoothie, page 142

PEACHES
How They Boost Brainpower: They're rich in water.

If you're having trouble focusing, eat a peach. Juicy peaches aren't just a sweet treat, they're packed with water. And given that your brain is 75 percent H_2O, slight dehydration can ruin your concentration and mood.

When researchers looked at the effects of varying levels of hydration on women, they found that a mild fluid deficit brought on headaches, soured their mental outlook, and impaired their ability to concentrate. If you're diabetic, about to have your period, or feeling under the weather, you're even more susceptible to the mood-lowering effects of dehydration.

➤ QUICK IDEA For a filling lunch salad, toss a sliced peach with 12 large cooked shrimp, 1 cup baby spinach, 1 sliced radish, and 1 tablespoon fresh lime juice. Season with a pinch of salt and ground black pepper.

➤ GOOD TO KNOW! Other water-packed produce: tomatoes, grapes, berries, and melon.

➤ SMART TIP When fresh peaches aren't in season, reach for canned. A 2013 study in the *Journal of the Science of Food and Agriculture* found the nutritional content of canned peaches to be similar to fresh peaches.

➤ BONUS! Peaches contain a special kind of polyphenol called chlorogenic acid, which may help prevent breast cancer.

———

RECIPE
◆ Peach Blueberry Smoothie, page 142

RED AND PURPLE GRAPES
How They Boost Brainpower: They're rich in anthocyanins.

Grapes are a prime source of anthocyanins, which are the pigments that give these fruits their red and purple color. Anthocyanins ramp up your brain's defenses against oxidative stress, a process that takes place when harmful compounds known as free radicals attack the cells throughout your body. Where do free radicals come from? They come from things like smoking, pollution, and even eating unhealthy foods. When free radicals strike your brain cells, it can make the cells slower and less efficient. As you get older, your body is less able to enlist antioxidants to undo the damage.

The same holds true for inflammation, which is basically your body's way of trying to repair injury. When cells are damaged by the wear and tear of daily life, they respond by producing anti-inflammatory proteins to restore the status quo. Yet, as the years pass, your body isn't as quick to respond. Anthocyanins help by rebooting your brain's anti-oxidant and anti-inflammatory defenses, so you're more likely to stay on your toes.

➤ GOOD TO KNOW! Red and purple grapes are also packed with pterostilbene, a plant chemical that improves—and may even reverse—age-related memory loss by stomping out oxidative stress.

➤ QUICK IDEAS Grapes can go savory. Fold them into curried whole-wheat couscous, sprinkle a handful into your next salad, or simmer them with red wine for a hearty sauce for roast chicken or pork.

➤ BONUS! These fruits supply resveratrol, the ingenious plant chemical that makes drinking red wine, in moderation, good for your heart.

➤ FACT A cup of grapes has about 100 calories.

———

RECIPE
◆ Carrots with Grapes and Dill, page 216

TUNA
How It Boosts Brainpower: It's rich in long-chain omega-3 fats.

Fat makes up a whopping 60 percent of your brain, where it plays an important role in mood, intellect, and memory. To function at its peak, your brain requires long-chain omega-3 fats like DHA and EPA, in particular (to learn even more about these healthy fats, turn to page 15 in chapter 2). A 2014 *Neurology* study found that women with the most omega-3s in their bloodstreams had larger brains than women with fewer omega-3s. More omega-3s were also linked to a bigger hippocampus, the part of the brain responsible for memory. But, since your body can't make them, you have to ingest them.

Now, scientists are learning that omega-3s from fish can help you stay sharp as early as your 40s. Dutch researchers queried 1,600 people ages 45–70 about their diets, then followed them for 5 years to see how they performed on tests of memory and mental speed. Their findings? Those who ate the most seafood outscored those who rarely touched it.

➤ **GOOD TO KNOW!** Since there's no formal recommendation on the exact amount of omega-3s you need to stay in top health, experts suggest eating at least two servings of fish a week.

➤ **QUICK IDEA** Pop open a can (or pouch) of tuna for one of your weekly fish meals. It's an easy way to bump up your omega-3 intake.

➤ **SMART TIP** Concerned about mercury? Stick with light tuna. It contains one-third of the mercury of white or albacore.

➤ **BONUS!** Three ounces of canned tuna give you an incredible 90 percent of your day's worth of brain-supporting B_{12} plus 17 grams of lean protein.

RECIPES
* Pepper-Crusted Tuna with Sesame Asparagus, page 192
* Tuna Fennel Wrap, page 156

WALNUTS

How They Boost Brainpower: They're rich in alpha-linolenic acid.

Walnuts are one of nature's best sources of the plant omega-3 fat alpha-linolenic acid, or ALA. In fact, walnuts boast more ALA than any other nut—and ALA, like long-chain omega-3 fats found in fatty fish, promotes brain health, in this case by keeping brain cell membranes flexible.

But there's an entirely different way walnuts do your brain good. They can help you get a better night's sleep. These nuts are one of the rare foods that contain melatonin, a hormone that regulates your body clock helping you slumber more soundly.

➤ **QUICK IDEA** In addition to walnuts, you can find melatonin in dried tart cherries. Toss together a couple of tablespoons of each for the ultimate evening snack.

➤ **GOOD TO KNOW!** Fourteen walnut halves contain 185 calories.

➤ **SMART TIP** Shelled walnuts can go rancid quickly, so store them sealed in your fridge. They'll stay fresh there for 6 months.

➤ **BONUS!** Like berries, walnuts are rich in brain-friendly polyphenols.

RECIPE
* Walnut-Crusted Chicken Cutlets, page 209

For brain-boosting

❍ Though you can't control every risk factor for Alzheimer's or depression, eating the right foods and getting plenty of rest and exercise are concrete steps you can take to improve your brain's health.

❍ To stay fueled all morning long, start your day with a breakfast that contains energizing complex carbs as well as slowly digested protein and fiber.

❍ Try to limit simple, processed sugars from soda and sweets.

❍ Aim for one serving of whole grains at every meal. It's an easy way to make half of your daily grains whole.

❍ Stay hydrated with water-filled fruits and vegetables, such as peaches, tomatoes, grapes, and berries.

❍ Focus on foods that increase the feel-good brain chemical serotonin, such as bananas and baked potatoes.

❍ If you're over 50, consider a senior-formula multivitamin for easily absorbed vitamin B_{12}.

❍ Keep an eye on your weight by watching portion sizes.

❍ Eat at least two servings of fatty fish a week to ensure you're getting sufficient brain-healthy omega-3 fats. If you don't eat fish, walnuts, chia seeds, canola oil, and flaxseeds can provide some of these beneficial fats as well.

❍ Don't forget to have fun! Engaging in challenging activities like games, puzzles, and reading, plus staying connected with friends and family, have been proven to help keep your brain young.

One-week brain-boosting meal plan

	BREAKFAST	LUNCH	DINNER
DAY 1	Peach Blueberry Smoothie*	Brown Rice Edamame Salad*	Spaghetti and Meatballs: Prepare 2 ounces whole-wheat spaghetti according to package directions. Top with 1/2 cup marinara sauce and 3 turkey meatballs. 2 cups tossed salad drizzled with 2 teaspoons extra virgin olive oil and 2 teaspoons balsamic vinegar
DAY 2	Gooey Strawberry French Toast*	Barley-Stuffed Pepper*	Soba Noodles with Shrimp, Snow Peas, Carrots, and Edamame*
DAY 3	Tropical Greek Yogurt Breakfast Parfait*	Black Bean Burger Salad*	Avocado Chicken* 1 medium baked potato with 2 tablespoons nonfat Greek yogurt or light sour cream 1/2 cup green beans sautéed in 1 teaspoon olive oil
DAY 4	PB & Banana Oatmeal*	Kale Salad with Chicken and Cheddar*	Pepper-Crusted Tuna with Sesame Asparagus* 1/4 cup brown rice, prepared according to package directions
DAY 5	1 cup bran flakes with 1 tablespoon chopped walnuts, 1/2 cup strawberries, and 1 cup 1% milk	Baked Potato "Burrito Bowl"*	Roast Pork Tenderloin with Blackberry Sauce* 1/4 cup whole-wheat couscous, prepared according to package directions 1/2 cup broccoli florets sautéed in 1 teaspoon olive oil
DAY 6	Better-for-You Blueberry Waffles*	Tuna Fennel Wrap*	Walnut-Crusted Chicken Cutlets* Carrots with Grapes and Dill* 1/4 cup quinoa, prepared according to package directions
DAY 7	Breakfast Burrito*	Couscous with Chickpeas*	Mediterranean Steak Salad*

*Recipe included in chapter 9

¾ cup grapes + 2 1-inch Brie cheese cubes

1 hardboiled egg sprinkled with curry powder
+ 8 small whole-grain crackers

Chia Pudding*
Cheesy Corn Tortillas*

Chocolate Chili Popcorn*

1 nut-based snack bar

12-ounce nonfat latte (6 ounces nonfat milk warmed in
the microwave + 6 ounces hot brewed coffee) + 1 peach

2 tablespoons peanuts (or other nuts) mixed with
2 tablespoons dried tart cherries

Pumpkin Smoothie*

1 sliced red pepper dipped in ¼ cup
hummus

PB & Banana "Sandwich"*

1 slice whole-wheat cinnamon raisin bread topped
with 2 tablespoons part skim ricotta

¾ cup edamame

6 ounces plain nonfat Greek yogurt with ¾ cup
blackberries

CHAPTER 6

Build Stronger Bones and Muscles

Women over 45 spend more days in the hospital on account of osteoporosis than for heart attacks, breast cancer, or diabetes. Avoid those unexpected doctor visits with these strength-boosting foods.

HOW YOUR BODY LOSES STRENGTH

Your bones may seem inactive, but they're actually living, dynamic tissue that's constantly being built up and broken down. Up until the age of about 25, your body is in peak bone-constructing mode, busily manufacturing bone tissue and replacing losses. However, by the time you reach middle age, the rate at which your bones are being dismantled begins to outpace the speed that they're rebuilt. Ditto for your muscles. Starting in your 40s, you shed about 1 percent of your muscle mass each year.

Think of your body as a house. Your bones are like the frame that keeps it upright, and your muscles are the bricks that make it solid. Like a home's frame and bricks can stand up

> TOP 8 RISK FACTORS
> ## *for osteoporosis*
>
> - Are over age 50 or postmenopausal
> - Have a family history of osteoporosis
> - Are thin or small-framed
> - Eat few fruits and vegetables
> - Have a diet low in calcium and vitamin D
> - Smoke
> - Drink too much alcohol
> - Are sedentary

the only way to keep your fortress strong. On the bone-building front, there's tried-and-true calcium as well as vitamin D. And now, new research is discovering that potassium, magnesium, and vitamin K also protect bones by helping to prevent fractures caused by osteoporosis and its precursor, osteopenia, or low bone mass.

➤ SMART TIP Weight-bearing exercise, like walking, hiking, jogging, weight lifting, dancing, and jumping rope, strengthens bones by making them work against gravity. For optimal bone health, aim for 30 minutes a day.

to the ravages of time and harsh weather for a a period of time until they inevitably start to weaken and buckle, your body also weakens over time. That's when it can become more difficult to do things like carry groceries from your car to the kitchen, walk the dog, or play with your children or grandchildren—unless you give your body a little TLC and preventive maintenance.

THE GOOD NEWS

It's not too late to change your fate! Researchers at the University of Texas Medical Branch recruited a group of older volunteers, around age 68, plus a group of teenagers to see how eating protein affects muscle building at different stages of life. They fed all of them lean burgers containing 30 grams of protein, and then measured the amount of muscle they manufactured. After comparing the results, they made an impressive discovery: Muscle synthesis increased equally for each group by a whopping 50 percent. But protein isn't

SUPER NUTRIENTS AND POWER FOODS
CALCIUM

What It Is: You have more calcium in your body than any other mineral. In addition to building and maintaining strong bones, calcium helps your muscles contract and relax, ensures your nervous system runs smoothly, contributes to proper blood clotting, and regulates blood pressure.

How It Keeps Bones Strong: Remember how bones are constantly being broken down and rebuilt? Well, there's a reason. Your bones and teeth are home to 99 percent of your body's calcium—they're like your body's calcium bank account. When you need calcium, for jobs like helping your heart beat or sending nerve impulses, you simply withdraw it from your bones. When you're young, this process works incredibly efficiently because dense bones provide a vast calcium stockpile. Once you reach your 40s—and you're no longer a bone-building machine—the picture changes.

Calcium is still withdrawn, but if it isn't regularly replenished, bones become fragile, brittle, and weak.

Healthy bone tissue looks like a honeycomb, with small regular spaces within a rock-solid framework. As bone density declines, those spaces that were once small and tight grow large and hollow, causing your bones to lose strength and fracture more easily. Osteoporosis literally means "porous bones." While consuming enough calcium can't change the fact that bone breaks down more quickly as you get older, it can ensure that you have plenty of the primary raw bone-forming material on hand, so your body can rebuild it faster.

➤ FACT In as little as 5–7 years after menopause, a woman can lose up to 20 percent of her bone density.

➤ GOOD TO KNOW! You need 1,000 milligrams of calcium a day until age 51. Then, you'll require 1,200 milligrams daily.

➤ DID YOU KNOW? Too much caffeine can cause you to lose small amounts of calcium. But adding 1–2 tablespoons of milk to your coffee or tea can reverse these losses, one Creighton University study found.

Where to Find It:
BOK CHOY

You may have heard that leafy green vegetables are a top source of calcium, but that's only half true. Certain leafy greens, like spinach, are high in oxalates, compounds that bind to calcium, making it difficult to absorb. To soak up the same amount of calcium found in one 8-ounce glass of milk, you'd have to eat 8 *cups*

THE TRUTH ABOUT
Calcium supplements

Forty-three percent of Americans, and 70 percent of older women, pop a daily calcium pill. Yet recent headlines that calcium supplements can boost the risk of heart disease may have you wondering if it's time to toss yours in the garbage.

For years, doctors and nutritionists recommended calcium supplements for bone health, especially for women who consume little dairy. Then, in 2010 a groundbreaking analysis of 15 studies that included 8,100 people linked consuming more than 500 milligrams of daily calcium from supplements to a 30-percent spike in heart attack risk. Despite this study's dramatic headlines, it's still not clear exactly how calcium might impair heart

health. To cloud matters further, a 2015 review of 18 studies and 63,500 women concluded that calcium supplements have no bearing on heart disease risk.

➤ BOTTOM LINE: Until there's more research on the subject, follow the lead of the American Heart Association, which recommends that people get their daily 1,000 to 1,200 milligrams-worth from naturally calcium-rich foods ("Eat Smart" on page 87 can show you the top choices). However, if you don't eat enough of these foods to meet your daily quota, talk to your doctor about a two-pronged approach of food plus supplements.

Squeeze more calcium into your day

Get your daily 1,000 to 1,200 milligrams of this Super Nutrient from a combination of these foods:

FOOD	SERVING SIZE	CALCIUM
Sardines	3.75 ounces	350 mg
Yogurt, nonfat plain	6 ounces	340 mg
Ricotta cheese, part skim	½ cup	335 mg
1% or fat-free milk	1 cup	300 mg
Calcium-fortified soy milk	1 cup	300 mg
Calcium-fortified tofu	½ cup	250 mg
Swiss cheese	1 ounce	220 mg
Mozzarella cheese, part-skim	1 ounce	220 mg
Canned salmon with bones	3 ounces	210 mg
Cheddar cheese	1 ounce	200 mg
Greek yogurt, nonfat plain	6 ounces	190 mg
Chia seeds	2 tablespoons	180 mg
Sesame seeds	2 tablespoons	175 mg
Parmesan cheese, grated	2 tablespoons	110 mg
Kale	1 cup raw, chopped	100 mg
Bok choy	1 cup raw, chopped	75 mg
Almonds	23 (1 ounce)	75 mg
Cottage cheese, 1% fat	½ cup	70 mg
Broccoli	1 cup cooked	60 mg

Select the best alternative milks

If you're lactose-intolerant or simply don't like the taste of cow's milk, there are lots of options to choose from. When shopping for alternative milks, just make sure they're unsweetened and fortified with at least 30 percent of the Daily Value for calcium, 25 percent of vitamin D, and—if you're a strict vegetarian or vegan—vitamin B_{12} (to learn more about B_{12} and vegetarian diets, see page 74 in chapter 5). Here's how the most popular kinds stack up nutritionally:

MILK*	CALORIES	PROTEIN	FAT	FIBER
1% cow's milk	100	8 g	2 g (1.5 g saturated)	0 g
Almond milk	30-50	1 g	2.5-3.5 g (0 g saturated)	1 g
Coconut milk beverage**	60	0 g	5 g (5 g saturated)	0 g
Hemp milk	70	3 g	5 g (0.5 g saturated)	2 g
Oat milk	130	4 g	2.5 g (0 g saturated)	2 g
Rice milk	90	<1 g	2.5 g (0 g saturated)	0 g
Soy milk	80	7 g	4 g (0.5 g saturated)	2 g

*All varieties are unsweetened.

**This kind of drink is lighter in fat, calories, and texture than traditional coconut milk in a can.

of cooked spinach. Not so with bok choy. This green—and many of its cruciferous friends, like broccoli and kale—isn't encumbered by oxalates. Just 1 cup of cooked bok choy packs as much calcium as half a glass of milk.

➤ QUICK IDEAS Swap in bok choy for lettuce in an Asian-style chicken salad, or for Chinese cabbage, asparagus, or green beans in your favorite stir-fry or noodle dish.

➤ BONUS! Bok choy is packed with other bone-supporting nutrients such as vitamins C and K and potassium.

RECIPES
◆ Beef Stir-Fry, page 160
◆ Sesame Salmon with Bok Choy, page 195

1% COTTAGE CHEESE
To get your daily dose of calcium, you'd have to drink more than 3 cups of milk. If that seems like a lot, try branching out with other dairy foods like cottage cheese. For about 160 calories, 1 cup of 1% cottage cheese gives you as much calcium as half a glass of milk plus a whopping 28 grams of protein.

➤ **QUICK IDEA** Pump up the calcium in your baked potato by mashing it with ½ cup of 1% cottage cheese.

➤ **GOOD TO KNOW!** Don't be confused by the "sell-by" date on the bottom of the package. While it's easy to assume this tells you the last date a food is safe to eat, it's actually a guide for supermarkets to know how long it's okay to display something on store shelves. Generally, cottage cheese is perfectly fine for up to 10 days after the sell-by date.

RECIPE
◆ Creamy Orange Banana Waffle, page 139

PROTEIN

What It Is: Protein is the raw material you need to build muscles. In addition, it forms tissues such as skin, bones, and organs as well as antibodies that fight disease, and hormones like insulin. You need it to make blood cells and for blood to clot properly as well.

You might remember from chapter 4 that your body produces protein from amino acids. There are 20 of them, to be exact. Of these, your body can make slightly more than half on its own. These are called nonessential amino acids since you don't need an external supply of them. The other half, known as essential amino acids, are found primarily in foods like chicken, steak, seafood, tofu, and dairy.

How It Keeps Muscles Strong: Beyond building muscle, protein ensures that you maintain it, too. When you lose muscle, strength is the first thing to go. But there are other more subtle issues that you can't see.

For instance, muscle's substantial weight puts pressure on your bones, helping them grow—and stay—big and thick. What's more, muscles are huge consumers of glucose and calories, greedily gobbling it up whenever you're moving. So when you lose muscle mass, you hinder the ability to efficiently regulate blood sugar and burn calories, making you more likely to become insulin-resistant and gain body fat.

While simply eating more protein helps a little bit, experts are now learning that

HOW MUCH PROTEIN DO YOU NEED IN A DAY?

You require about 0.5 gram of protein for every pound you weigh, specifically:

IF YOU WEIGH	YOU NEED THIS MUCH PROTEIN EACH DAY
110 pounds	55 grams
120 pounds	60 grams
130 pounds	65 grams
140 pounds	70 grams
150 pounds	75 grams
160 pounds	80 grams
170 pounds	85 grams
180 pounds	90 grams
190 pounds	95 grams
200 pounds	100 grams

Beans—they're what's for dinner!

Canned beans are the ultimate healthy convenience food. Keep your pantry stocked with lots of different kinds, and you'll always have a base for a healthy meal on hand.

TYPE OF BEAN	TRY IT IN
Black	Tacos, burritos, quesadillas, vegetarian chili, black bean soup, such as Black Bean Tomato Soup (recipe on page 150)
Cannellini	Minestrone, pasta marinara, white-bean chili, salads such as Quinoa Cannellini Salad (recipe on page 154)
Chickpeas	Hummus, vegetable stews, falafel, salads, such as Couscous with Chickpeas (recipe on page 151)
Kidney	Meat, chicken, or turkey chili; three-bean salad
Lentils	Curries, lentil soup, salads,
Pinto beans	Tacos, burritos, quesadillas, meat, and vegetarian chili

the amount you eat at *each* meal may be as important as the quantity you consume in a day. Unlike carbs or fat, your body can't store protein. If you down more than you need, the rest is either burned for fuel or—if you've eaten enough—stored away as fat. How much is enough, and how much is too much? It depends on your body size (see "How Much Protein Do You Need in a Day?" on page 89), but the ideal amount for most women is somewhere between 20 and 30 grams per meal. That's the amount in 3–4 ounces of grilled chicken or salmon.

If you take the time to make sure you're spacing your protein evenly throughout the day—at breakfast, lunch, and dinner—the payoffs are tremendous. A study conducted at the University of Texas Medical Branch found that people who consumed 30 grams of protein at every meal built 25 percent more muscle than when they ate the same amount of protein distributed into portions of 11 grams at breakfast, 16 for lunch, and 63 at dinner.

➤ DID YOU KNOW? When you diet, you don't just lose fat, you shed muscle, too. New research reveals that eating more protein when you're cutting calories can help you hold on to that muscle. In a 2012 study, researchers put people on a calorie-restricted diet with either 0.75 gram or 0.36 gram of protein for each pound they weighed. The results: even though weight loss was similar between both groups, women in the higher protein group lost more fat while retaining more muscle than their lower-protein counterparts.

Where to Find It:
CANNELLINI BEANS

When it comes to bone health, a growing body of research reveals that the foods you eat, day in and day out, are a major contributor to how strong—or weak—your bones are. When Australian researchers compared several different eating patterns, they found that people who favored a diet with loads of refined grains, processed meats, and sodas had the flimsiest bones. On the other hand, those who gravitated toward a regimen similar to the Mediterranean diet—filled with beans, vegetables, seafood, nuts, seeds, and rice— had the sturdiest frames. That beans are high in bone-friendly nutrients like protein, potassium, and magnesium may help explain it. Mild, chameleon-like cannellinis work well in pastas, soups, and salads, so they make an especially useful pick.

➤ SMART TIP Canned beans are a speedy alternative to cooking and soaking dried beans. Choose no-sodium-added canned varieties, as too much sodium can raise blood pressure (read more about sodium and blood pressure on page 19 in chapter 2). If your supermarket doesn't stock these, rinsing and draining regular canned beans washes away 40 percent of their sodium.

➤ QUICK IDEA Mash rinsed and drained no-salt-added canned cannellini beans with a squirt of lemon juice for a protein-packed spread for whole-grain crackers.

➤ FACT One cup of these beans gives you 17 grams of protein and 11 grams of fiber.

➤ GOOD TO KNOW! Tofu, chia, and quinoa also provide protein with less saturated fat and more fiber than meat, chicken, fish and dairy.

➤ BONUS! As noted, cannellini beans are rich in potassium and magnesium (you can learn more about potassium on page 19 in chapter 2 and magnesium on page 32 in chapter 3 as well as on pages 98 and 99 later in this chapter). A cup contains 21 and 35 percent of your daily quota of each, respectively.

————

RECIPE
◆ Quinoa Cannellini Salad, page 154

EGGS

Eggs boast one of the highest-quality forms of protein available, meaning that your body soaks it up more readily than proteins from other kinds of foods, from beef to soy.

Just one large egg provides 6 grams of protein for only 75 calories. What's more, eggs are rich in a special amino acid called leucine, which helps build muscle.

➤ FACT Most people eat only one-third as much protein at breakfast as they do at dinner.

➤ QUICK IDEA Give your eggs a protein boost by scrambling them with a few tablespoons of lowfat cottage or ricotta cheese.

➤ DID YOU KNOW? Thanks to improved methods of feeding chickens, today's eggs contain 185 milligrams of cholesterol. That's 14 percent less than in 2002. Eggs are also surprisingly low in fat, with just 5 grams of total fat and 1.5 grams of saturated fat per large egg.

➤ SMART TIP If just one egg seems too small, scramble one whole egg with two whites, and you'll get the volume and protein of two scrambled eggs—and still keep cholesterol in check.

➤ GOOD TO KNOW! Tempted to simply scramble all the whites and toss the yolks entirely?

Add protein to your breakfast

Eggs aren't your only option. These speedy meals do the trick:

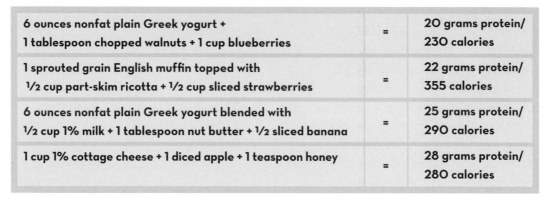

6 ounces nonfat plain Greek yogurt + 1 tablespoon chopped walnuts + 1 cup blueberries	=	20 grams protein/ 230 calories
1 sprouted grain English muffin topped with ½ cup part-skim ricotta + ½ cup sliced strawberries	=	22 grams protein/ 355 calories
6 ounces nonfat plain Greek yogurt blended with ½ cup 1% milk + 1 tablespoon nut butter + ½ sliced banana	=	25 grams protein/ 290 calories
1 cup 1% cottage cheese + 1 diced apple + 1 teaspoon honey	=	28 grams protein/ 280 calories

Don't. The yolk contains over half of each egg's protein plus the bulk of the nutrients such as vitamins A and D plus iron. Most health experts agree that one egg a day is perfectly safe for most people, though if you have heart disease or diabetes, speak with your doctor.

RECIPES
- ◆ Breakfast Burrito, page 138
- ◆ Huevos Rancheros, page 140
- ◆ Sardine, Cucumber, and Endive Sandwich, page 155
- ◆ Spinach-Feta Omelet, page 144

PART-SKIM RICOTTA CHEESE
One quarter cup of part-skim ricotta gives you 7 grams of protein for only 85 calories. And ricotta doesn't supply just any type of protein. Ricotta is the best source of whey protein around. Why does whey protein matter? Like eggs, whey is rich in the muscle-building amino acid leucine. In fact, ricotta has nearly four times as much leucine as milk and more than twice as much as yogurt.

➤ SMART TIP When buying ricotta, stick with part-skim varieties. Nonfat types can be rubbery, while the whole-fat version has at least 60 percent more total and saturated fat than part-skim.

RECIPES
- ◆ Apricot Ricotta Breakfast Sundae, page 137
- ◆ Better-for-You Blueberry Waffles, page 137
- ◆ Cantaloupe Breakfast Bowl, page 138
- ◆ Pomegranate-Apricot Breakfast Crostini, page 143
- ◆ Spaghetti with Beets, Greens, and Ricotta, page 201
- ◆ Ziti with Eggplant and Ricotta, page 210

YOU MAY NEED EXTRA VITAMIN D IF YOU:

◆ Are black or Hispanic

◆ Have a body mass index, or BMI, of 30 or more

◆ Are pregnant or nursing

◆ Have osteoporosis, osteomalacia, or rickets

◆ Have chronic kidney disease

◆ Have problems absorbing certain nutrients due to conditions such as celiac disease, Crohn's disease, or ulcerative colitis

◆ Have had gastric bypass surgery

◆ Have been diagnosed with hyperparathyroidism

◆ Take corticosteroids or take certain medications for weight loss or to lower cholesterol

◆ Have a history of bone fractures

VITAMIN D

What It Is: Unlike other nutrients, your body has the unique ability to make vitamin D from a special form of cholesterol in your skin. When the sun's UV rays hit your skin, they transform this compound to a precursor of vitamin D, which is later transported to your liver and then to your kidneys, where it is converted to the active form of vitamin D known as vitamin D_3.

Just 10 minutes of sunshine two or three times a week between the hours of 10 a.m. and 3 p.m. can give you all the D you need during the summer. But in most parts of the country during the fall, winter, or spring, the sun's rays simply aren't strong—or abundant—enough to help you make the vitamin D you need. Plus, when it's cold out, most people don't spend enough time outdoors to soak up the UV rays needed to make sufficient amounts of this nutrient. Sunscreen is important for preventing skin cancer, yet that can interfere with your ability to make vitamin D, too. Combine all of that with the fact that very few foods actually contain this vitamin, and it's no wonder 42 percent of Americans are vitamin D deficient.

That's why it couldn't hurt to ask your doctor to test your levels of vitamin D to find out *exactly* how much is right for you, as

Get the vitamin D you need

Even if you have a stellar diet, vitamin D can be hard to come by. You can drink it in fortified milk, but you'd have to down nearly 1.5 quarts a day to get the 600 IU most women require. Similarly, you could eat fatty fish like salmon, halibut, and trout every day, though that would likely grow monotonous. Of course, soaking up 10 minutes of sunshine two or three times a week can boost your level of vitamin D. The downside: it's not always safe for your skin. To make sure you're completely covered each day, aim for a combination of vitamin D-rich foods plus a vitamin D_3 supplement, the form of vitamin D that's fully active so it's easiest for your body to use (check out the "Nutritionist's Note" on page 93 for tips on when to take your pill).

levels can vary widely from person to person. If you fall into any of the groups below, you may need to consider a supplement (see the "Nutritionist's Note" on page 93 for some handy advice).

How It Keeps Bones Strong: When it comes to sturdy bones, calcium and vitamin D work together as a team. Even though you need calcium to build up your skeleton, you can't absorb it without its helper vitamin D. Fall short, and bones become frail, increasing your risk of osteoporosis. But vitamin D isn't just about your bones. It keeps your immune system in top shape, ensures proper cell growth, and fights inflammation, too. Health experts are also finding that it's crucial for strong muscles. When researchers at the University of Massachusetts at Amherst and the University of Connecticut looked at the relationship between vitamin D and muscle strength, they found that people with the healthiest vitamin D levels had the most powerful arms and legs.

➤ **DID YOU KNOW?** The older you get, the harder it is to make vitamin D, as you produce less of the special form of cholesterol your body uses to synthesize vitamin D from sunlight.

➤ **GOOD TO KNOW!** Vitamin D is measured in units known as international units (IU). You need at least 600 IU of vitamin D a day until age 71. After that, minimum requirements increase to 800 IU. That said, many experts feel these may not be sufficient and that 1,000 IU is a better goal.

➤ **SMART TIP** Your body must have fat to absorb vitamin D, so make sure to take yours at mealtime.

Where to Find It:
SARDINES
Nature's best sources of vitamin D are fatty fish like tuna, salmon, and sardines. One 3.75-ounce can of sardines gives you a hefty 30 percent of your day's vitamin D and, thanks to their bones, more calcium than a glass of milk.

But vitamin D and calcium aren't the only reasons to stock up on these little fish.

Sardines are also rich in omega-3 fats, believed to protect against inflammation. You may remember from chapter 2 that inflammation is a kind of damage that occurs when your body tries to respond to an injury. Just as inflammation can harm your arteries, it can also accelerate bone breakdown. Sardines are such bone-building powerhouses that a 2011 *American Journal of Clinical Nutrition* study found that eating three or more servings a week of them and other dark fish (think mackerel or salmon) was linked to denser thighbones.

> ➤ **QUICK IDEA** Toss sardines into pasta marinara for a fast vitamin D and calcium fix.
> ➤ **SMART TIP** Like tuna, sardines come canned in either water or oil. If you prefer yours packed in oil, be sure to drain them well so that they're not swimming in it. Whenever possible, opt for no-added-salt sardines to cut down on sodium.
> ➤ **DID YOU KNOW?** You can also get vitamin D from fortified foods like milk, orange juice, and some brands of cereal plus small amounts from eggs.

RECIPE
◆ Sardine, Cucumber, and Endive Sandwich, page 155

FOOD LABEL SLEUTH
Vitamins and minerals

When you scan the nutrition facts label of your favorite food, you may wonder why you see certain vitamins and minerals listed and not others. Right now, food companies are only required to reveal nutrients that many of us don't get enough of (like vitamin D, calcium, iron and potassium) and those we eat too much of (like sodium). So, just because, say, vitamin B_6 and zinc aren't included on the box, that doesn't mean they're not inside.

Of the nutrients that do appear, you'll find them listed as a percentage of the Daily Value (refresh your memory on the Daily Value on page 8 in chapter 1). Those in excess of 20 percent are outstanding.

VITAMIN K
What It Is: Like vitamin D, vitamin K is a fat-soluble vitamin, meaning your body requires fat from foods to absorb it. While most of the K you eat comes from leafy green vegetables like kale, broccoli, and Swiss chard, the bacteria in your digestive system can also synthesize small amounts.

How It Keeps Bones Strong: Vitamin K's biggest role is helping blood clot properly. Its name even comes from the German word *koagulation*. It has another job, too: it keeps your bones strong by binding special proteins to calcium. Researchers at Tufts University queried nearly 900 elderly volunteers about their intake of vitamin K–filled foods and then tracked them for 7 years. At the end of the study, they found that those with the highest vitamin K intake (around 250 micrograms daily, compared to the basic 90 micrograms

What's the difference between fat-soluble and water-soluble vitamins?

They're absorbed and stored differently.
Specifically, certain nutrients dissolve in either water or fat—but not both. As a result, fat-soluble vitamins, namely A, D, E, and K, are easily stored in your fat tissues, so you don't need to eat them every day. Water-soluble vitamins, such as vitamin C and the B vitamins, require water to dissolve, so they can't be stored in fat tissue. Because your body doesn't hold on to these for very long, pay extra attention to consuming them every day.

you need each day) were two-thirds less likely to suffer hip fractures than those whose diets contained the least.

➤ **GOOD TO KNOW!** You also require vitamin K for healthy cartilage, the layer of connective tissue that covers and protects joints and bones (think knees and elbows). Without enough of this buffer, you can develop arthritis.

➤ **FACT** Twenty-seven million Americans have arthritis. One study found that people with low vitamin-K levels were 33 percent more likely to have arthritis in one or both knees.

➤ **DID YOU KNOW?** Vitamin K can interfere with the action of certain blood thinners. If you're taking blood-thinning medication,

speak to your doctor before increasing your intake of vitamin K-rich foods.

Where to Find It:
KALE
This green vegetable boasts more vitamin K than any other food—472 micrograms per cup. Like bok choy and broccoli, kale is also rich in a form of calcium that's easy to absorb. If that wasn't enough, it dishes up plenty of magnesium, vitamin C, and potassium, too.

➤ **QUICK IDEA** For a vitamin K boost, thinly slice kale and toss it into tomato, vegetable, or minestrone soup.

➤ **SMART TIP** Whether it's lettuce, spinach, watercress, or kale, almost all salad greens are loaded with vitamin K, so aim for at least one serving of salad a day.

➤ **SMART TIP** While green leafy vegetables are the best sources of vitamin K, you can rack up

JUST DON'T LIKE KALE?

If the taste of kale is too strong for you, try baby kale. It's mild and tender like baby spinach. What's more, research reveals that *all* kinds of green vegetables (from broccoli and leafy greens to zucchini and peppers) are smart food for your skeleton, as they're usually packed with vitamin K, potassium, and magnesium. (And some—like kale—are good sources of calcium, too.) One study found that women who ate green or yellow vegetables every day were five times less likely to have low bone mass than women who didn't down a daily serving.

10 percent of your daily dose (or more) from 1 tablespoon of soybean or canola oil.

RECIPE

- ◆ Kale Salad with Chicken and Cheddar, page 153

PARSLEY

Vegetables aren't the only way to rack up your vitamin K. One quarter cup of chopped parsley gives you nearly three times your daily allotment of this nutrient. It's also a surprising source of vitamin C with ¼ cup chopped delivering 27 percent of your daily dose. No time to clean and chop it? Dried parsley as well as basil, thyme, and sage contains respectable amounts of vitamin K, too.

➤ **QUICK IDEA** Add a handful of fresh parsley to salads for a bright, peppery flavor.

➤ **GOOD TO KNOW!** You can store fresh parsley in the refrigerator for up to 5 days. Simply wash, dry, and wrap it in a paper towel. Then store it in a plastic bag in the crisper.

RECIPES

- ◆ Lemon Shrimp, page 181
- ◆ Linguine with Tomatoes, Spinach, and Clams, page 183
- ◆ Quinoa Cannellini Salad, page 154
- ◆ Slow Cooker Chicken Marbella, page 198

OTHER STRENGTHENING POWER FOODS

BEETS

How They Make You Stronger: They're rich in nitrates.

If you'd like to work out longer with less effort, these root vegetables could make that wish come true. Beets are rich in nitrates, compounds that have been shown to increase production of nitric oxide, or NO. NO, as you may remember from chapter 2, enhances blood flow (to learn more, turn to page 25). A growing body of research is now finding that NO's circulation-promoting abilities also improve endurance. In a 2012 Saint Louis University study, volunteers ate roughly four beets or an equal amount of cranberry relish. Then, 75 minutes later, they participated in a 5K run, a great weight-bearing exercise. Not only did the beet group run faster than the placebo group, they also reported feeling less fatigued during the first mile of the run.

➤ **QUICK IDEA** Beet greens make a tasty swap for spinach. Mix them into salads or sauté with garlic and olive oil and serve as a side dish.

➤ **GOOD TO KNOW!** Lettuce, spinach, bok choy, cabbage, and carrots are naturally rich in nitrates, too.

➤ **SMART TIP** If you've ever cooked beets before, you know they can take a long time. Make things easier by picking up canned or precooked vacuum-sealed beets. Slice them and stuff into a roast beef sandwich or toss them into a Waldorf salad.

RECIPES

- ◆ Beet Tabbouleh with Grilled Chicken, page 162
- ◆ Spaghetti with Beets, Greens, and Ricotta, page 201

CASHEW NUTS

How They Make You Stronger: They're rich in magnesium.

Magnesium plays many important roles in your body, such as regulating blood pressure and heart rate. It's also critical for strength. More than half of the magnesium in your body is in your bones, making them dense and heavy. The other half lives in your muscles and tissues, where it helps your muscles contract.

Since most women don't eat enough of this nutrient in their diets, nuts like cashews are especially beneficial. Just 1 ounce provides 74 milligrams of magnesium, or 23 percent of your daily requirement.

➤ **SMART TIP** Nut butters like cashew, peanut, and almond butter are all good sources of magnesium. Keep a jar of one (or each!) on hand for sandwiches, toast, or whole-grain crackers, or as an indulgent topping for your morning oatmeal.

➤ **BONUS!** One ounce of cashews serves up 70 percent of your day's worth of copper, a mineral needed to build collagen (learn how collagen improves strength on page 100).

RECIPE
◆ Cashew-Chicken Stir-Fry, page 164

CURRY POWDER

How It Makes You Stronger: It's rich in curcumin.

Curry powder isn't one spice—it's a blend of up to 20 different spices. One of these is turmeric, which gives curry its dazzling yellow-orange color. Turmeric boasts a secret ingredient: curcumin, a powerful antioxidant that fights the inflammation that can cause arthritis. One study found that the compound is so effective that it relieved arthritis-related knee pain almost as well as certain pain medications.

➤ **QUICK IDEA** Whisk a dash of curry powder into equal parts Greek yogurt and mayo. Then toss with diced hard-cooked eggs for a spiced-up egg salad.

➤ **BONUS!** Curry powder's turmeric may help prevent Alzheimer's disease.

———

RECIPE
◆ Curried Chickpea Pita, page 152

GOOD NITRATES VS. BAD NITRATES

You may be wondering why nitrates from vegetables are good while nitrates from processed meats spell trouble. Right now, experts are wrestling with the same question. What they do know is that nitrates from vegetables don't seem to increase cancer risk, likely due to their ample supply of cancer-fighting antioxidants, phytonutrients, and fiber. Another factor may be that, unlike nitrates from vegetables, nitrates from processed meats latch on to amino acids in your digestive system, forming carcinogenic compounds. So, while it's still prudent to avoid processed meats, nitrate-rich vegetables continue to be natural health foods.

Cola cravings

If nothing quenches your thirst like an ice-cold soda pop, it could be doing a number on your bones. Cola contains phosphoric acid, a food additive that gives cola its tart flavor. The trouble is that phosphoric acid also pulls calcium out of your bones and limits calcium absorption. In fact, people who drink just one cola a day have bones that are up to five and a half percent weaker than those of people who don't drink cola. If you're hooked, but would like to drink less, try these tricks:

◆ **Cross it off your shopping list.** Yes, it's obvious, but if there's no cola in your house, you can't drink as much of it.

◆ **Upgrade to iced tea.** Freshly brewed tea has been linked to stronger bones, thanks to a cast of bone-supporting nutrients including fluoride, phytoestrogens, and flavonoids.

◆ **Think small.** If you're not ready to break up with cola for good, cut back by pouring yours into a smaller glass. Or buy those sleek 7.5-ounce cans that you've seen on store shelves. You'll down 40 percent less cola and cut out 50 calories per can.

◆ **Ice it down.** Before you go cold turkey, you may need to wean yourself off your favorite drink's flavor (and caffeine). Dilute it by filling your cup to the top with ice before you pour.

◆ **Get your bubble fix elsewhere.** You may not be craving cola's taste as much as its carbonation. Try swapping in fizzy mineral water (or club soda) with a wedge of orange or lemon. If you're wondering about other kinds of flavored soda, you may want to bypass those, too. A 2014 Harvard School of Public Health study found that each daily soda (not necessarily cola) a woman drinks can raise her risk of hip fracture by 14 percent.

DRIED PLUMS

How They Make You Stronger: They're rich in potassium.

Whether you call them prunes or dried plums, these chewy fruits can keep your skeleton in top shape. Just six dried plums serve up as much potassium as a banana. And potassium doesn't get nearly enough credit for its role in bone support. Here's why: eating too many refined carbohydrates, meat, cheese, and soft drinks has been shown to weaken bones. These foods increase acid levels in your blood after you eat them. To quickly bring blood acid levels back down to normal levels, your body steals calcium from your bones, as calcium helps neutralize acid. Over time, those calcium losses add up and can weaken your frame. Enter potassium, which lowers blood-acid levels in the same way that calcium does.

➤ QUICK IDEA For a satisfying snack, cut one piece of reduced-fat string cheese into quarters. Slice open four dried plums and stuff each with a piece of cheese.

➤ SMART TIP Puréed dried plums are an easy way to lower fat in baked goods like muffins, quick breads, and brownies. Simply combine 1 ⅓ cups dried plums with 6 tablespoons hot water. Then purée and swap in for half the butter or oil called for in the recipe. You'll reduce fat by up to 30 percent!

➤ **BONUS!** Dried plums give you vitamin K. Six provide 34 micrograms of the nutrient, or 38 percent of your daily fill.

DRIED TART CHERRIES
How They Make You Stronger: They're rich in antioxidants.

It's hard to motivate yourself to go to the gym when your muscles are sore and tired. You could pop some ibuprofen, or you could nibble on dried tart cherries instead. These dried treats are packed with antioxidants like flavonoids and anthocyanins, which quash post-exercise inflammation that can cause muscles to ache.

Tart cherry juice also does the trick. Several studies report that it reduces post-race muscle soreness in runners and may help after pumping iron as well. When college students drank 12 ounces of tart cherry juice twice daily, they experienced less muscle pain after muscle-strengthening exercises than those who sipped a placebo. While 24 ounces of juice a day might be a little much (unless you're a marathon runner), adding ½ cup to your smoothie may help.

➤ **GOOD TO KNOW!** Don't be fooled by the "tart" in tart cherries. They're actually intensely sweet, so try a handful to satisfy your next sweet tooth.

➤ **DID YOU KNOW?** Other than walnuts, dried tart cherries are one of the few foods that contain the sleep-inducing hormone melatonin.

KIWI
How It Makes You Stronger: It's rich in vitamin C.

You know that vitamin C can help you bounce back from a cold. But did you know it's also good for your skeleton? Vitamin C is critical in forming collagen, a protein that's the foundation of bone. When you build bone, the first step is to lay down scaffolding made of collagen. Once that infrastructure is in place, minerals like calcium and magnesium are deposited to fill it in, making it hard and fracture-resistant. Since collagen is one of the raw materials your body uses to construct tendons and ligaments, it also keeps bones stable. You can get plenty of collagen-building vitamin C from citrus fruits like oranges and grapefruits, but don't forget about kiwis. Just one of these little green fruits serves up nearly an entire day's worth.

➤ **SMART TIP** Cutting a kiwi in half and scooping out the flesh with a spoon is the easiest way to eat it.

➤ **BONUS!** Kiwis are high in vitamin K. One kiwi gives you 31 percent of your daily dose.

For stronger bones and muscles

○ Consuming sufficient calcium is one of the best things you can do to keep your bones strong. Aim for at least 1,000 milligrams of calcium daily (1,200 if you're 51 or older) from a combination of lowfat dairy (or milk alternatives), leafy greens, dark fish (such as salmon or sardines), and calcium-fortified foods.

○ If you don't eat dairy products, talk to your doctor about a calcium supplement.

○ Aim for at least 1,000 IU of vitamin D_3 each day from a combination of food and supplements. If you take a supplement, every night at dinner is the easiest and best time.

○ Aim to eat 20–30 grams of protein at each meal.

○ Eat at least five servings of fruits and vegetables daily. Of these, make sure to include at least one serving of leafy greens.

○ Cook with fresh and dried green herbs for extra vitamin K.

○ Limit alcohol to one drink a day, as excessive alcohol consumption can weaken bones.

○ Take a brisk walk or make sure to do some kind of weight-bearing exercise for about 30 minutes every day. It's an easy way to keep bones and muscles strong!

One-week meal plan for stronger muscles and bones

	BREAKFAST	LUNCH	DINNER
DAY 1	Spinach-Feta Omelet* 12-ounce nonfat latte (6 ounces nonfat milk warmed in the microwave + 6 ounces hot brewed coffee)	BBQ Turkey Burger* 1 cup grape tomatoes	Spaghetti with Beets, Greens, and Ricotta*
DAY 2	Gooey Strawberry French Toast*	Mediterranean Pasta Salad*	Steak and Onion Tacos with Fresh Tomato Salsa* Ambrosia Parfaits*
DAY 3	1 cup high-protein whole-grain breakfast cereal with two chopped dried plums and 1 cup 1% milk	Quinoa Cannellini Salad*	Slow Cooker Chicken Marbella* 1 cup cooked string beans drizzled with 1 teaspoon olive oil and 1 teaspoon balsamic vinegar
DAY 4	Apricot Ricotta Breakfast Sundae*	Curried Chickpea Pita*	Cashew-Chicken Stir-Fry* 2 mini dark chocolate bars
DAY 5	Huevos Rancheros*	Apple Spinach Salad*	Sesame Salmon with Bok Choy* ¼ cup brown rice, prepared according to package directions
DAY 6	Tropical Greek Yogurt Breakfast Parfait*	Kale Salad with Chicken and Cheddar*	Ziti with Eggplant and Ricotta*
DAY 7	Creamy Orange Banana Waffle*	Sardine, Cucumber, and Endive Sandwich*	Beet Tabbouleh with Grilled Chicken* 1 cup mixed berries

*Recipe included in chapter 9

Unlimited veggies dipped in ¾ cup nonfat plain yogurt mixed with a large pinch of curry powder

17 cashew nuts

Chia Pudding*

¾ cup edamame

1 hardboiled egg drizzled with Sriracha hot sauce + 8 small whole-grain crackers

6 ounces nonfat plain Greek yogurt with ½ cup blueberries

Strawberry Smoothie*

Chocolate Chili Popcorn*

PB & Banana "Sandwich"*

2 kiwis + 12-ounce nonfat latte (6 ounces nonfat milk warmed in the microwave + 6 ounces hot brewed coffee)

1 apple and 2 1-inch Brie cubes

Spicy Trail Mix*

1 nut-based snack bar

1 warmed corn tortilla topped with ¼ cup warmed black beans and 1 tablespoon salsa

PART TWO

TURN BACK THE CLOCK FOR A YOUNGER-LOOKING YOU

CHAPTER 7

Help Skin Look It's Youngest

In the last 15 years, the number of women using Botulinum toxin to smooth wrinkles has skyrocketed 703 percent. Want a less invasive way to minimize lines? Meet your new Power Foods.

HOW SKIN AGES OVER TIME

By the time you reach menopause, you may notice that your skin is drier and less supple than it used to be. But did you know that these changes start to occur as early as your 20s? Around that time, skin's production of collagen and elastin, supportive proteins that keep it firm and elastic, slows down. At the same

time, sebaceous glands in your skin begin to secrete less sebum, a wax-like substance that's a natural moisturizer.

Lifestyle makes a difference, too. Staying out of the sun and covering up with sunscreen are fundamental, as are choosing not to smoke, limiting the amount of alcohol you drink, and even exercising more. Also, the foods you eat go a long way in preserving your skin's youthful appearance—or not. One 2007 *American Journal of Clinical Nutrition* study of 4,025 women between the ages of 40 and 74 reported that those who consumed too much of certain nutrients, namely carbohydrates, had older-looking skin. Eating just 50 additional grams of carbohydrates a day— roughly the amount in three slices of white bread—increased skin thinning and wrinkling by more than a third.

As with blood sugar or brain-related concerns (in chapters 3 and 5, respectively), where those carbs come from is important. If they're from sweets, such as soda, syrup-flavored lattes, brownies, or cookies, wrinkles may form even faster. When you eat—or drink—too much sugar, it builds up in your bloodstream faster than your cells can use it. This excess sugar then attaches to collagen and elastin, forming stiff, inflexible structures called advanced glycation endpoints (AGEs) that make skin cells rigid. Because skin no longer flexes with ease, fine lines and wrinkles develop.

And sugar isn't the only culprit. High-heat cooking such as frying can also spur formation of AGEs. For instance, a French fry has nearly 90 *times* more of these aging compounds than a boiled potato. Fry an egg, and you'll generate 60 times as many AGEs as you would from boiling it. While this doesn't mean you can never enjoy a cookie or an onion ring, avoiding sugary and fried foods as often as possible could help slow visible signs of aging.

THE GOOD NEWS

Just as nutrients from food are continually delivered to your heart, brain, and bones,

---

YOU ASKED
Is dairy making my skin break out?

Maybe. Studies show that drinking milk, especially skim milk, is a mild acne trigger. And pimples aren't only an issue for teenagers. Twenty-six percent of women ages 31–40 and 12 percent of those between the ages of 41 and 50 said they still suffered from breakouts, according to a 2012 *Journal of Women's Health* study. Experts aren't sure why milk makes some people's skin break out. But they suspect that it may increase the production of hormones, such as IGF-1, that stimulate excessive sebum secretion, promoting breakouts. If you have a stubborn case of acne, limiting dairy products might be worth a try. If you do, remember to get plenty of calcium from a combination of nondairy calcium-filled foods (you can find them listed on page 87 in chapter 6) plus supplements, if necessary.

---

they're also transported to your skin. Many are even stored within your skin's layers, feeding, hydrating, and protecting it from environmental insults like pollution and the sun's damaging light. In the pages that follow, you'll read all about how certain Super Nutrients and Power Foods improve your skin.

Before you do, it's helpful to learn a little bit about the skin's structure. Your skin is made of three basic layers. On the top is the epidermis, a protective coating that locks in

How to up your fluid intake

If you know you should drink more water, but never really do, you can still get the fluids you need with these simple suggestions:

◆ **Start your day with a smoothie.** Who says you have to eat your breakfast? Smoothies deliver loads of fluids and several servings of produce in one shot. Make yours more filling by adding a little healthy fat from avocados, flax seeds, or chia seeds.

◆ **Or try oatmeal.** Oats might start out dry, but once cooked in water, oatmeal is 84 percent fluid. Toss in some fresh berries, and you'll gain even more fluids.

◆ **Eat yogurt.** Weighing in at 85 percent water, one 6-ounce container of yogurt nets 5 ounces of H_2O.

◆ **Slurp soup.** Broth-based soups are an easy way to pump up your fluids. Just bear in mind that some soups can be high in sodium, so opt for reduced-sodium varieties.

◆ **Try coffee or tea.** Contrary to what you may have heard, caffeinated drinks don't dehydrate you. Instead, when you drink a caffeinated drink it acts like a mild diuretic, causing you to lose a small percentage of its fluid. That's why the Institute of Medicine says that caffeinated drinks can still help you meet your fluid needs. So, if a hot steaming mug of coffee or a glass of iced tea is your preference, that's okay.

moisture and shields against foreign invaders such as germs. Below the epidermis lies the dermis, a thicker cushion that supports and nourishes the epidermis. Finally, the dermis rests on the hypodermis, a foundation of fat and additional collagen, which holds in heat and keeps you safe from injury.

If your mother always told you that eating too many greasy foods would ruin your complexion, she was only partially right. Eating enough fat—and the right kind of it—can actually improve your skin's appearance (for more on healthy fats, see page 11 in chapter 2). Fat is in every layer of your skin, from the top epidermis all the way down to the innermost hypodermis, providing moisture, nourishment, and cushioning. It's so important that one study found that women with plenty of fat in their food had skin that was more supple and elastic than women who favored a lowfat diet.

One more factor that it's easy to overlook: water. Fluids keep skin cells plumped and hydrated, plus they cleanse away impurities. However, as you age, your sense of thirst becomes less keen, so drinking up is key.

➤ **GOOD TO KNOW!** A recent Scottish study found that eating roughly four servings of fruits and vegetables a day provides nutrients known as carotenoids (such as beta-carotene), which give skin a golden glow that's healthier and more radiant-looking than a suntan. But don't limit yourself to four servings. For optimal health overall, experts recommend a minimum of five daily servings of produce.

➤ **FACT** When researchers compared the skin of people over the age of 40 who exercised to those who didn't work out, they found that regular exercisers had complexions that resembled those of people in their 20s and 30s.

SUPER NUTRIENTS AND POWER FOODS
LYCOPENE

What It Is: Lycopene is a plant pigment that gives produce like tomatoes, watermelon, pink grapefruit, guava, and papaya their rosy color. It's also a powerful antioxidant that helps prevent prostate cancer and may defend against cancers of the lung and stomach. Like vitamins A, D, E, and K, lycopene is fat-soluble (for more on fat-soluble nutrients and how they work, go to page 96 in chapter 6). That means it can accumulate in your body's fat tissues, providing a prolonged supply to nourish your skin.

How It Helps Skin Look Its Youngest: Whether you tend to tan or burn, it's easy to see the immediate effects of the sun on your skin. What's not as obvious is the damage brewing beneath the surface. There, UV light generates free radicals, toxic molecules that ambush your DNA (to learn more about this process, known as oxidation, flip to page 14 in chapter 2). In your skin, free radicals attack collagen. Over time, that can cause collagen to weaken and break down, encouraging wrinkles and furrows to set in.

Lycopene is a powerful antioxidant that can protect your skin from sun damage. German researchers divided volunteers into two groups, feeding one 2 teaspoons of olive oil and the other 2 teaspoons of olive oil plus 2 ½ tablespoons of tomato paste each day. After 10 weeks, they treated the volunteers' skin with powerful UV light. When they compared the results from each group, they found that the tomato paste eaters experienced an impressive 40 percent less sun damage to their skin than the olive oil group.

➤ SMART TIP You don't need to drench your food in fat to absorb its lycopene. About 1 teaspoon of olive or canola oil will do the trick.

WAIT, AREN'T TOMATOES A FRUIT?

Tomatoes live a double life as a fruit and a vegetable. Botanically, they are a fruit, the part of a plant that grows from a flower. At the same time, produce that's served as part of a meal can also be called a vegetable, which is how the USDA classifies tomatoes. So pick your definition, and go with it.

When it comes to lycopene, the kind from canned tomatoes or tomato sauce could be even better for you than fresh tomatoes. Canning tomatoes or making tomato sauce requires heat, which breaks down lycopene into a form that's easier for your body to absorb. Just watch the level of salt in your canned tomatoes and opt for low- or no-sodium varieties. Along with raising your blood pressure, sodium can cause fluid to accumulate around your eyes, making them puffy and swollen.

➤ QUICK IDEAS Work more lycopene into your day by tossing pink grapefruit sections with avocado and endive, drizzling ripe heirloom tomatoes with extra virgin olive oil, or sprinkling crushed macadamia nuts on top of papaya slices.

Where to Find It:
TOMATOES

Right now, you probably have fresh tomatoes sitting on your counter, marinara sauce in your fridge, and tomato paste in your pantry. Americans eat so many tomatoes that they're the second most popular vegetable in the United States, right behind potatoes. They're also the number one source of lycopene.

➤ SMART TIP You don't have to spend a fortune at your local juice bar to get the nutrition your skin craves. A small can of low-sodium vegetable juice is brimming with lycopene, plus vitamins A and C.

➤ QUICK IDEAS Don't just save tomato sauce for pasta. Spoon it onto eggs, baked potatoes, or broccoli for an instant lycopene fix.

RECIPES
- Black Bean Tomato Soup, page 150
- Broccoli and Tomato Pizza, page 150
- Corkscrew Pasta with Sausage and Fennel, page 172
- Garlic Shrimp and Swiss Chard on Polenta, page 176
- Linguine with Tomatoes, Spinach, and Clams, page 183
- Slow Cooker Italian Lentil and Vegetable Stew, page 199
- Steak and Onion Tacos with Fresh Tomato Salsa, page 206

YOU ASKED
I've heard jarred marinara sauces are packed with added sugars. Should I avoid them?

No. While it's true that many brands of marinara sauce have some added sugar, that doesn't mean you should cross them off your shopping list. A half cup of marinara sauce gives you about 1 ¾ teaspoons of sugar. Some of this is natural, as tomatoes, like most produce, contain their own sugars (about ¾ teaspoon per medium tomato). The rest is added.

Even still, the amount of sugar in marinara is a fraction of what you'd get from regular cola, sweetened lattes, or cookies. Case in point: A 12-ounce can of soda serves up 10 teaspoons of sugar, roughly six times as much as you'd get from the marinara. In exchange for a small amount of sugar, you'll gain vitamins A, E, and K, as well as lycopene. The amount of sugar does vary from brand to brand, though, so be sure to compare labels. Or try cooking up your own tomato sauce with the easy recipe for Summer Tomato Sauce on page 220 in chapter 9.

- Summer Tomato Sauce, page 220
- Ziti with Eggplant and Ricotta, page 210

PAPAYA

Papaya is a yummy way to eat more lycopene. But that's not the only reason to enjoy this tropical fruit. One cup of papaya offers your entire daily dose of collagen-building vitamin C and provides 10 percent of vitamin A, another skin-supporting vitamin you'll read about later in this chapter. In addition to keeping your complexion firm and smooth, papayas are rich in papain, an enzyme that helps break down protein, so they're a natural digestive aid as well.

➤ **QUICK IDEA** For a 10-minute meal, serve slices of papaya and avocado with grilled shrimp and a squirt of lime juice.

➤ **SMART TIP** Papayas are fully ripe when their skin is orange-yellow. If yours is still green, you can help it ripen faster by storing it in a paper bag.

RECIPE

◆ Sunrise Smoothie, page 144

VITAMIN A

What It Is: As discussed in chapters 2 and 4, some nutrients come in two different forms, one from plant foods and another from animal foods. For instance, there's heme iron from meat and non-heme iron in vegetables and grains. Or long-chain omega-3 fats like DHA and EPA in fatty fish versus shorter-chain ALA from plants like flax and chia. There are also two forms of vitamin A. The first type, known as preformed vitamin A, is in foods like milk, meat, and fish. Like EPA, DHA, and heme iron, it's fully active as soon as you eat it. Plant vitamin A is more like non-heme iron or ALA. Found as a combination of alpha-carotene, beta-carotene, and beta-cryptoxanthin in green leafy vegetables and yellow-orange produce, your body must covert these to vitamin A before they can be used. Similar to lycopene, both vitamin A and these substances, known as carotenoids, are fat-soluble, so it's important to eat them with some fat for absorption.

➤ **GOOD TO KNOW!** When you buy foods like frozen spinach or carrots, you won't see the amount of alpha- or beta-carotene or beta-cryptoxanthin on the Nutrition Facts panel. Instead you'll find it included in the Daily Value for vitamin A, which includes the amount of vitamin A that your body converts from these carotenoids.

How It Helps Skin Look Its Youngest: Vitamin A works throughout your body to support special epithelial cells. On the inside, epithelial cells form the protective mucous membranes that coat your mouth, sinuses, lungs, intestines, stomach, uterus, and more. Outside, they make up your skin, helping your epidermis seal out moisture (so skin doesn't become waterlogged) and nourishing cells lower down in the dermis. This vitamin also shields your skin from UV damage, and beta-carotene scavenges your skin for free radicals that can cause premature aging.

➤ **GOOD TO KNOW!** Just because some is good, more isn't necessarily better. Too much preformed vitamin A can weaken bones. If you take a multivitamin, check the label to make sure yours provides no more than 5,000 IU of vitamin A, of which half should come from beta-carotene.

On organic produce

When you see a food labeled organic, it's easy to assume that it's better for you. But that's not always the case. Just like conventional foods, there are healthy organic foods and organic junk foods such as cookies, chips, and even candy.

In the case of produce, organic fruits and vegetables do provide the benefit of being raised without pesticides and fertilizers, but they can be pricey, and that's not always practical. The higher cost of organic produce can make it difficult to get the 4 cups of produce you need daily for optimal health. That's why I believe the benefits of eating lots of conventional produce outweigh the cost of going organic. However, if you're concerned about pesticides and fertilizers in your food, you can try a targeted strategy of buying mostly conventional produce and selectively purchasing organic versions of fruits and vegetables that conventionally contain the most pesticides, such as apples, strawberries, grapes, celery, and peaches. For a full list of the highest and lowest pesticide produce, visit the Environmental Working Group's website, http://www.ewg.org/foodnews/list.php#. And, of course, wash or rinse fruits and vegetables before eating them.

Where to Find It:
CARROTS

These root vegetables are prime sources of alpha- and beta-carotene. They're so rich in beta-carotene that this plant chemical was named in their honor. That makes them vitamin A powerhouses—with 73 percent of your daily quota in one carrot. And if you've ever been on a low-carb diet that forbade carrots because they were supposedly packed with sugar, you'll be happy to learn that one carrot contains less than 3 grams of natural sugar (read more about natural sugars on page 39 in chapter 3). As far as carbohydrates go, carrots have roughly 6 grams each plus 2 grams of digestion-slowing fiber. Glycemic index–wise, carrots weigh in at a low 35 (check out page 33 in chapter 3 for info on the glycemic index). So munch away!

➤ **QUICK IDEA** Next time you make coleslaw, pump up the vitamin A by mixing equal parts store-bought shredded carrots and cabbage.

➤ **SMART TIP** After you buy carrots, cut off the tops, then store them in a plastic bag. They'll stay fresh in your fridge for 2 weeks.

➤ **BONUS!** A *British Journal of Dermatology* study found that foods rich in beta-carotene, especially carrots, may protect against psoriasis, an autoimmune skin condition that affects more than 7 million Americans.

RECIPES
- Apple Spinach Salad, page 147
- Brown Rice Edamame Salad, page 151
- Carrots with Grapes and Dill, page 216
- Cauliflower Mac 'n' Cheese, page 168
- Curried Chickpea Pita, page 152

- Soba Noodles with Shrimp, Snow Peas, Carrots, and Edamame, page 200
- Spice-Roasted Chicken, Red Onions, Carrots, and Parsnips, page 204

SWEET POTATOES

With more vitamin A and beta-carotene than any other vegetable, one medium sweet potato delivers more than one and a half times your daily vitamin A. It gives you close to one third of your day's vitamin C, too. But sweet potatoes aren't just about the vitamins. They're also an impressive source of fiber, a nutrient that whisks impurities out of your system for a clearer complexion. One sweet potato provides 4 grams. That's as much as you'd get from 1 cup of oatmeal.

➤ QUICK IDEA Blend ½ cup of cooked sweet potato into your next smoothie. In addition to supplying skin-friendly nutrients, it will keep you full longer!

➤ DID YOU KNOW? Even though we often call sweet potatoes yams and vice versa, they're not the same vegetable. Yams come from an entirely different plant and contain substantially less vitamin A and beta-carotene.

➤ GOOD TO KNOW! Sweet potatoes can be orange, purple, or even white. Deeper-orange varieties contain the most beta-carotene, while purple ones are full of anthocyanins, nutrients that improve brain health (page 79 in chapter 5 can tell you how).

RECIPE
- Slow Cooker African Sweet Potato–Peanut Stew, page 196

SWISS CHARD

Eating 1 cup of sautéed Swiss chard gives you more than three quarters of your daily dose of vitamin A. Plus, this vegetable is loaded with beta-carotene, vitamins C and E, and fiber. When Japanese researchers measured the moisture and elasticity of 716 women's skin, they found that those who ate the most green and yellow vegetables had the fewest crow's-feet.

➤ QUICK IDEAS If you've never eaten Swiss chard before, it makes a delicious alternative to spinach. Remove the ribs and stalks, and sauté the leaves. You can also add chard to omelets, frittatas, and pasta.

➤ SMART TIP After you've cut out the ribs and the stalks, don't throw them out. Simply sauté, steam, or grill them like asparagus, then drizzle with a little extra virgin olive oil and a dusting of sea salt for a tasty side dish.

➤ BONUS! Swiss chard is an outstanding source of vitamin K, a nutrient that helps keep bones strong. One cup cooked chard contains six times your daily fill.

———

RECIPE
- Garlic Shrimp and Swiss Chard on Polenta, page 176

VITAMIN C

What It Is: Along with keeping your immune system strong and fighting infection, vitamin C is a powerful antioxidant that mops up free radicals throughout your body. Unlike the other skin-friendly nutrients you've read about in this chapter, vitamin C is water-soluble, so you don't need to eat it with fat to absorb it. However, since your tissues can store only limited quantities, it's essential to make sure you get your fill every day.

How It Helps Skin Look Its Youngest:
Even though your body can't store much vitamin C, small amounts do accumulate in the skin, where it stimulates collagen formation. Chapter 6 explained that collagen is the foundation of healthy bones. It's the glue that cements skin cells together as well. When you have a cut or a scrape, collagen mends torn cells. It also fights signs of aging by keeping your skin pliable and firm. Without enough, skin becomes rough, dry, and chapped, and cuts can take a longer time to heal.

As you get older, though, your skin becomes less efficient at holding on to collagen-boosting vitamin C. And the sun can deplete your vitamin C even more. The same is true if you smoke or live with someone who does.

➤ **FACT** A study published in the *American Journal of Clinical Nutrition* found that women with the most vitamin C in their diets were less likely to have dry skin or wrinkles than those who consumed the least.

➤ **GOOD TO KNOW!** You require 75 milligrams of vitamin C a day. But if you smoke or live with a smoker, you need an extra 35 daily milligrams.

Where to Find It:
BROCCOLI
Just 1 cup of cooked broccoli provides 135 percent of your daily vitamin C. And broccoli may even improve your skin color, thanks to beta-carotene. Beyond that? Researchers are now finding that the vegetable may fend off skin cancer, too. That's because broccoli contains the plant chemical glucoraphanin, shown to shield against UV damage.

➤ **BONUS!** Broccoli contains special plant chemicals known as glucosinolates that naturally flush toxins from your body. See page 53 in chapter 4 to learn more about how they work.

➤ **SMART TIP** Even though broccoli is a potent foe against skin cancer and other forms of the disease, heat destroys many of its cancer-fighting nutrients. Try yours raw in a broccoli slaw or a tomato, broccoli, and cannellini bean salad.

————

RECIPES
◆ Broccoli and Tomato Pizza, page 150
◆ Cashew-Chicken Stir-Fry, page 164

MANGOS
A mango a day could keep wrinkles away—given that 1 cup provides at least three quarters of your daily requirement for vitamin C and 13 percent of A. But there's more: mangos contain other plant compounds that may increase collagen production and lessen fine lines, according to a 2013 Korean study.

➤ **GOOD TO KNOW!** If you're trying to figure out if a mango is ripe, don't rely on its color. Instead, give it a gentle squeeze. If it yields slightly, it's ready to eat.

➤ **QUICK IDEA** Skewer mango chunks and shrimp, brush with lime juice and canola oil, and grill 5–6 minutes.

HOW TO CUT A MANGO

1 Stand a mango lengthwise on a cutting board.

2 Place knife ¼ inch from the center on one side and try to locate the large pit in the middle. Once you do, slice along the pit through the fruit, to release one of its "cheeks." Repeat on the opposite side.

3 Cut long vertical slices in each cheek, taking care not to cut through the skin. Rotate the cheek 90 degrees and cut horizontal slices to form a cubed pattern.

4 From the skin side, push the mango flesh inside out and gently remove the mango chunks with a knife.

Source: The National Mango Board

➤ **SMART TIP** Keep a bag of frozen mangos on hand to blend into smoothies or to defrost and stir into yogurt.

➤ **GOOD TO KNOW!** Mangos are low in pesticide residues. Other produce that's low in pesticides includes asparagus, onions, frozen peas, corn, and avocados.

➤ **BONUS!** Mangos are rich in lupeol, an antioxidant that may protect against skin cancer.

RECIPE
- Spiced Pork Tenderloins with Mango Salsa, page 202

VITAMIN E

What It Is: This fat-soluble vitamin lives in your cells' outer membranes, waiting to pounce on free radicals before they ever have the chance to harm your cells' interior. However, sometimes vitamin E needs a little help from its friend vitamin C. The reason: once vitamin E neutralizes free radicals, it loses its antioxidant powers. But like a set of jumper cables that give new life to a dead car battery, vitamin C gives vitamin E an antioxidant jump-start, so it can get back to the business of fighting free radicals.

How It Helps Skin Look Its Youngest: No nutrient works harder to keep your skin healthy than vitamin E. For starters, it's the most plentiful antioxidant in your skin, defending against sun damage by absorbing UV light, rendering the rays less likely to mar DNA and break down collagen. This nutrient is also a natural moisturizer, stimulating the production of hydrating sebum in your sebaceous glands. And it works quickly: adding more vitamin E–rich foods to your plate can increase sebum production in as little as a week.

➤ **FACT** Most Americans don't get all the vitamin E they need, at 15 milligrams a day. Since it's found mostly in nuts, seeds, and oils, you're especially likely to fall short if you don't eat much of their healthy fat.

➤ **GOOD TO KNOW!** High doses of vitamin E can thin your blood. While you can't get too much from foods, steer clear of high-dose supplements, especially if you take blood thinners.

➤ **BONUS!** Vitamin E keeps your heart healthy and may protect against dementia and macular degeneration, too.

Where to Find It:
ALMONDS

These nuts are a top source of hydrating vitamin E. Just 1 ounce, or about 23 almonds, gives you half of the E you need in a day. Like vitamin C, skin levels of vitamin E can be depleted by exposure to sunlight. Your skin's vitamin E also declines with age, so it's especially important to meet your daily quota as you get older.

➤ QUICK IDEA Toss a handful of almonds on your morning cereal. In addition to moisturizing your skin, their healthy fat will help you stay full until lunchtime.

➤ GOOD TO KNOW! Spinach is also rich in vitamin E. A cup of cooked spinach gives you 26 percent of your day's worth.

➤ DID YOU KNOW? Almonds may be lower in calories than previously believed. A recent study in the *American Journal of Clinical Nutrition* found that 1 ounce contains 129 calories instead of the 164 calories originally estimated.

➤ BONUS! With roughly two and a half times as much calcium as walnuts and pistachios, almonds have more calcium than any other tree nut, at 75 milligrams per ounce.

———

RECIPES
* Maple Almond Oatmeal, page 141
* Orange and Apricot Quinoa, page 141
* Tropical Greek Yogurt Breakfast Parfait, page 145

OTHER SKIN-HEALTHY POWER FOODS
CANTALOUPE
How It Helps Skin Look Its Youngest: It's rich in water.

If you go through more moisturizer than you'd care to admit, you might want to try a little hydration from the inside out. Your skin is 64 percent water, so even a little bit of dehydration can make you look parched. While you should aim for about 90 ounces of fluid a day, 20 percent (or roughly 18 ounces) can come from water-filled foods. Make cantaloupe, which is 90 percent water, one of your go-tos.

➤ QUICK IDEA For a 100 percent fruit popsicle, insert popsicle sticks into peeled cantaloupe wedges and freeze.

➤ SMART TIP Wash cantaloupe (and any fruit) just before you cut it to remove potentially harmful bacteria from the skin.

➤ BONUS! One cup of this juicy melon dishes up nearly three-quarters of your daily need for skin-enhancing vitamin C plus 39 percent of your daily dose of vitamin A.

———

RECIPES
* Cantaloupe Breakfast Bowl, page 138
* Cantaloupe Cucumber Salad, page 215

DARK CHOCOLATE
How It Helps Skin Look Its Youngest: It's rich in flavonoids.

Go ahead, pinch yourself. Dark chocolate is *good* for your skin. Made from cocoa, chocolate contains flavonoids, the same family of antioxidant plant chemicals that fight cancer. Now, experts are learning that, in the right amounts, cocoa flavonoids offer multipronged skin protection by absorbing damaging UV light, shielding against free radicals, and boosting blood flow that delivers nutrients. To see just how powerful flavonoids might be, researchers divided women into two groups: One sipped a daily cocoa drink that contained as many cocoa flavonoids as 3.5 ounces of dark chocolate. The other women downed a less-potent cocoa beverage. After 12 weeks, the women in the high flavonoid group had skin that was smoother, plumper, and less sun-damaged than those who drank the less-potent concoction.

➤ **GOOD TO KNOW!** When shopping for cocoa, look for non-alkalized varieties. They contain more flavonoids than alkalized, or Dutch process, cocoa.

➤ **SMART TIP** Cacao nibs are made from the inside of cocoa beans, which are used to make chocolate and cocoa powder. Toss some cacao nibs into yogurt or oatmeal for an antioxidant boost. Along with their flavonoid punch, they're surprisingly high in fiber at 2 grams per tablespoon.

➤ **QUICK IDEA** For a cocoa flavonoid kick, stir a spoonful of unsweetened cocoa into your morning or afternoon coffee.

RECIPES
- Chocolate Chili Popcorn, page 224
- Good-for-You Hot Chocolate, page 225

DARK MEAT CHICKEN

How It Helps Skin Look Its Youngest: It's rich in iron.

After decades on the diet *don't* list, dark meat chicken is finally back on the menu. Dark poultry is especially rich in iron, a mineral that gives your complexion a pink glow. Without enough, you can end up looking pale and sallow. And one skinless drumstick sports only 1 gram of saturated fat and 4.5 grams of total fat. In exchange, you'll get high-quality heme iron that your body can use quickly and efficiently—all for about 150 calories.

➤ **SMART TIP** For faster thawing, individually wrap drumsticks or put them in separate zip-top bags. Then spread them on a baking sheet and defrost overnight in the fridge.

➤ **DID YOU KNOW?** The skin on your chicken isn't as evil as you've been led to believe. One drumstick with skin only contains about 2 more grams of saturated fat than a drumstick that's skin-free, according to the USDA's National Nutrient Database.

RECIPES
- Slow Cooker Chicken Marbella, page 198
- Spice-Roasted Chicken, Red Onions, Carrots, and Parsnips, page 204

SAFER CHICKEN PREP

Lots of people think they should rinse chicken before cooking it. But rinsing raw chicken is actually *more* likely to cause food poisoning by spreading its bacteria through splashing. So transfer chicken directly from package to pan, or prepare yours on a separate cutting board designated for meat products only. After cooking, make sure your chicken is safe to eat by using a meat thermometer to test for an internal temperature of 165°F.

ROMAINE LETTUCE
How It Helps Skin Look Its Youngest: It's rich in water and vitamin A.

With 95 percent of its weight coming from water, these crunchy greens are an ingenious way to sneak in extra fluids. Plus, 1 cup of shredded romaine provides 29 percent of your daily vitamin A. It also contains nitrates, nutrients that can improve endurance during exercise (turn to page 97 in chapter 6 to learn more). With only 8 calories per cup, these leaves could also be the world's biggest calorie bargain.

➤ SMART TIP If you store apples in your fridge, keep in mind that they release ethylene gas that can turn lettuce leaves brown. So store romaine as far away as possible from them, or keep apples in a plastic bag.

➤ QUICK IDEA For a new spin on salad, try grilled romaine. Simply slice one romaine head in half lengthwise, mist with cooking spray, and sear on the grill for about 4 minutes, flipping halfway. Remove from heat, chop, and add it to your salad just like raw romaine.

➤ GOOD TO KNOW! Prewashed bagged lettuce can be a huge time-saver. Yet, even though it's been cleaned, it can still contain unsafe bacteria, so be sure to give it a good rinse before you use it.

RECIPES
* Black Bean Burger Salad, page 149
* Grilled Shrimp Caesar, page 152

SUNFLOWER SEEDS
How They Help Skin Look Its Youngest: They're rich in linoleic acid.

Sunflower seeds boast more linoleic acid than just about any other food—just ¼ cup provides more than two thirds of your daily quota. Linoleic acid, or LA, is one of the most plentiful polyunsaturated fats in the epidermis, where it's a key component of your skin-cell membranes. It's also important in the dermis below that. There, it thwarts inflammation that can lead to uncomfortable conditions like psoriasis.

As a natural moisturizer, LA keeps skin hydrated. But your body can't manufacture it, so you have to get it from food. Case in point: when British researchers looked at the skin of 4,025 women, they found that those who ate more linoleic acid–rich foods were at least 22 percent less likely to have dry, thinning skin.

➤ QUICK IDEA Sprinkle toasted sunflower seeds and microwaved frozen peas into warm basmati rice for healthy fats, filling protein, and fiber.

➤ SMART TIP If you're concerned about nut allergies, sunflower seeds and sunflower butter are an easy way to add nut-like flavor and beneficial fats to your food.

➤ GOOD TO KNOW! Sunflower seeds turn rancid quickly, so make sure to store them in the fridge.

➤ BONUS! One quarter cup of sunflower seeds gives you 82 percent of your day's vitamin E.

RECIPES
* Crunchy Sunflower Butter Sandwich, page 139
* Pomegranate-Apricot Breakfast Crostini, page 143

One-week meal plan for younger skin

	BREAKFAST	LUNCH	DINNER
DAY 1	Maple Almond Oatmeal*	Grilled Shrimp Caesar*	Spiced Pork Tenderloins with Mango Salsa* ¼ cup quinoa, prepared according to package directions 1 cup broccoli drizzled with 2 teaspoons olive oil
DAY 2	Cantaloupe Breakfast Bowl*	Black Bean Tomato Soup*	Slow Cooker African Sweet Potato–Peanut Stew*
DAY 3	Breakfast Burrito*	Salmon Pesto Sandwich* Cantaloupe Cucumber Salad*	Spice-Roasted Chicken, Red Onions, Carrots, and Parsnips* 1 cup mixed berries
DAY 4	Pomegranate Apricot Breakfast Crostini*	Apple Spinach Salad*	Soba Noodles with Shrimp, Snow Peas, Carrots, and Edamame* 1 cup papaya chunks
DAY 5	Sunrise Smoothie*	Veggie Burger Parmesan*	Garlic Shrimp and Swiss Chard on Polenta*
DAY 6	Spinach-Feta Omelet* topped with ½ cup marinara sauce	Quinoa Cannellini Salad*	Cashew-Chicken Stir-Fry* 2 ½-inch pineapple slices sprayed with nonstick cooking spray and grilled on each side for 3 minutes
DAY 7	Crunchy Sunflower Butter Sandwich*	Broccoli and Tomato Pizza*	Grilled Chicken Salad with Avocado and Grapefruit* ½ cup rinsed and drained canned black beans, warmed

*Recipe included in chapter 9

1 ounce dark chocolate
Ambrosia Parfait*

12-ounce nonfat latte (6 ounces nonfat milk warmed in the microwave + 6 ounces hot brewed coffee) + 2 kiwis
¾ cup edamame

PB and Banana "Sandwich"
1 sliced red bell pepper dipped in 1 tablespoon tahini

Good-for-You Hot Chocolate*
23 almonds

Unlimited broccoli and cauliflower florets dipped in your favorite tomato salsa.
6 ounces nonfat vanilla Greek yogurt sprinkled with 1 tablespoon sunflower seeds

Pumpkin Smoothie*
1 piece part-skim mozzarella string cheese + 1 apple

Chocolate Chili Popcorn*
6 ounces nonfat plain yogurt with 1 cup sliced strawberries

CHECKLIST
For skin rejuvenating

❍ A produce-filled diet is one of the best steps you can take for younger-looking skin. Aim for at least five servings a day. Since colors are an indicator of skin-friendly carotenoids, try to include as many hues as possible, especially red, yellow, orange, and green.

❍ Too much preformed vitamin A from supplements can weaken bones. If you take a daily multivitamin, make sure it contains no more than 5,000 IU of vitamin A, of which half should come from beta-carotene.

❍ Staying hydrated ensures that your skin stays plump and moist. Keep a bottle or pitcher of water on your desk or kitchen counter and toss another bottle in your bag for when you're out and about. Eating water-packed produce helps, too.

❍ Remember, healthy fat is your skin's friend. Focus on the kinds from whole foods like nuts, seeds, extra virgin olive oil, and fatty fish.

❍ If you're prone to stubborn outbreaks, consider a dairy-free diet. But be sure to include plenty of nondairy calcium sources or take a supplement.

❍ Save sugar-sweetened drinks and foods like cookies, cakes, and brownies for a special treat.

❍ Don't forget to look for added sugars on the Nutrition Facts panel of food packages.

❍ Try to avoid fried foods by baking, boiling, or sautéeing instead.

❍ Lifestyle matters! So steer clear of cigarettes, limit time in the sun, and try to squeeze in 30 minutes of exercise every day.

CHAPTER 8

Better Hair, Nails, and Teeth

*Surprise: 40 percent of those with thinning hair are women.
As you age, your nails and teeth can suffer, too.
These protein- and mineral-rich foods are here to help.*

HOW YOUR HAIR CHANGES OVER TIME

Your hair has such a powerful impact on your emotional outlook that volunteers in a Yale University study said simply thinking about a bad hair day deflated their self-confidence. And even though the right styling tools and hair care products can make the difference between so-so and fantastic strands, there are other factors that affect your hair, including your overall health, genes, and fluctuating hormones (swings in estrogen levels after childbirth or during menopause temporarily cause hair to shed).

But after you enter your 40s, you may notice some more permanent changes in your hair's fullness and texture. The reasons for this are twofold: first, the number of hairs you grow begins to decline, plus each individual hair becomes thinner in diameter. As your scalp starts to produce less sebum, or oil, hair can become drier and frizzier.

The proper foods and nutrients can go a long way in helping you grow or maintain thicker, glossier hair. Take protein—hair growth requires a *lot* of it. Yet, when it comes to doling out protein, your body is stingy, parsing it out first to the organs and cells that need it most for survival. Because hair has no other real function than to keep you warm, it's fairly far down on the list of priorities. As a result, if you're not consuming enough protein, hair growth can become sluggish (for more on exactly how much protein you need each day, flip to page 89 in chapter 6). The same holds true for calories: your body requires energy for new growth, which is why hair loss is a common side effect of crash diets.

OTHER CAUSES OF HAIR LOSS

- ◆ An over- or underactive thyroid
- ◆ Iron-deficiency anemia
- ◆ Oral contraceptives
- ◆ Blood thinners, antidepressants, and blood-pressure–lowering medications
- ◆ Surgery or illness

➤ GOOD TO KNOW! In addition to treating skin conditions, dermatologists are experts in hair and nails. If you've been struggling with thinning hair or weak nails, a visit to the dermatologist could help.

HOW YOUR NAILS AND TEETH CHANGE OVER TIME

Just as your hair changes over time, so do your

THINNING HAIR COULD BE A SIGN OF HEART TROUBLES

When men lose their hair, it often (although not always) follows a predictable pattern, receding at the hairline and slowly inching backward. This type of hair loss, known as male pattern baldness, is usually caused by a combination of genetics and hormones. In women, those same factors can cause a condition known as female pattern hair loss. (You may have seen this if you've ever noticed a friend with an unusually wide part or scanty hair growth on top of her head.) For decades, health experts have known that men with male pattern baldness are more prone to heart disease. Now, they're finding that women with female pattern hair loss are predisposed to heart troubles, too. When researchers investigated this relationship, they found that women with female pattern hair loss were 26 percent more likely to suffer from coronary artery disease. While you may not be able to change your genes, if it runs in your family, you can protect your cardiovascular health by eating a heart-smart diet (turn to chapter 2 to find out how).

nails. When nail growth slows, nails become drier and more brittle—in fact, 20 percent of adults have brittle nails. Whether it's from washing dishes or cleaning the house with harsh detergents, women's nails tend to take more of a beating than men's, so be sure to use rubber gloves for an added layer of protection. And even though your manicure may make your nails look nicer for the short term, nail polish removers and polishes also parch your nails, making them more prone to peeling and chipping.

As the years pass, you may notice subtle changes in your smile, too. The first is the color of your teeth, which can become darker and stained from colas or cups of coffee or tea. While that's just cosmetic, you may also become more prone to something you thought was only a problem for kids—tooth decay. The reason? The older you become, the more medications you're likely to take. And many of these can make your mouth dry, reducing the amount of saliva available to wash away bacteria that can lead to tooth decay. Because your gums naturally begin to recede, tooth sensitivity may become an issue as well.

THE GOOD NEWS

Remember the last time you got a bad haircut? Even though you hated it, you knew it would grow out…eventually. Your hair and nails are continually in a state of renewal. In 1 year you'll sprout 6 inches of new hair, and in half that time, you'll produce an entirely new set of fingernails.

In chapter 7, you learned about nutrients that help your skin look its youngest. You might have noticed that many of these were vitamins. On the pages that follow, you'll read about a lot of minerals—especially iron, zinc, and silicon—that can help your hair and nails stay strong and healthy (for more about the differences between vitamins and minerals, see the "Nutritionist's Note" on page 124). But don't expect a hair- and nail-friendly diet to work its magic overnight. Their health mirrors your diet over the past 6 months or even longer. Remember, the benefits you'll get from eating the Power Foods in this chapter can take a while to show. In the meantime, keep in mind that these beauty foods have other perks, such as giving you more energy,

YOU ASKED

Can too many processed foods make my hair thin?

Not exactly. However, a less-than-stellar diet might cause it to thin, especially if it's robbing your hair of vital nutrients and causing you to gain extra pounds. Weight gain can lead to something called metabolic syndrome, a cluster of five conditions including too much belly fat, low HDL cholesterol, high blood pressure, elevated triglycerides, and elevated blood sugar. Not only does metabolic syndrome boost your risk of diabetes, heart disease, and stroke, new research finds that it may cause male pattern baldness and female pattern hair loss. It's also been linked to psoriasis of the scalp.

helping you slim down, and keeping you healthier overall.

When it comes to your smile, there's even more happy news: your teeth aren't nearly as likely to show signs of age as your hair and nails are. You've no doubt heard that avoiding sugary foods and sodas can help keep your smile its best—well, so can eating targeted foods such as cheese and yogurt that actually fight cavities. Bothered by staining and yellowing? There are foods—especially those rich in fiber—that can scrub stains from your teeth, making them whiter and brighter.

SUPER NUTRIENTS AND POWER FOODS
IRON

What It Is: Iron is an essential part of hemoglobin, a protein in red blood cells that ferries oxygen throughout your body, keeping cells energized. Oxygen also keeps your immune system strong, promotes healing, and helps remove impurities from your system.

But your iron requirements change substantially as you age. From your teens until your late 40s or early 50s, you'll lose iron every month when you get your period, which is why premenopausal women require more than twice as much iron as women who have gone through menopause. During pregnancy, requirements increase even more, skyrocketing by an additional 50 percent to expand blood volume and support a growing baby. That can make consuming enough of this mineral a challenge. However, without sufficient iron, your body can't get the oxygen it needs, making you tired, listless, and unable to concentrate. Later in life, when menopause kicks in and monthly blood loss is no longer an issue, iron needs shrink, making getting the iron you need fairly easy.

How It Keeps Hair and Nails Healthy: Take a close look at your nails. Are the beds nice and pink? That's a sign that you're eating plenty of iron. If you were to fall short, the skin beneath would become pale—much in the same way a lack of iron can wash out your complexion. More severe iron deficiency can take an even greater a toll on your nail health, changing their shape and causing them to sink inward, a condition experts call "spoon nails."

Iron also helps your hair by supplying oxygen to your hair follicles, small pockets in your scalp that grow individual strands of hair. When iron levels dwindle, the follicles can't function properly and hair begins to fall out. And iron deficiency may be an even bigger culprit in shedding prior to menopause than it is later on in life. In one study, Korean dermatologists compared the iron levels of pre- and post-menopausal women who were seeking treatment for hair loss. While low iron didn't have much of an impact on the older women, it was significantly linked to a sparser head of hair in premenopausal patients.

➤ **FACT** Before age 51 (when most women will have reached menopause), you require 18 milligrams of iron a day. After that, once you're no longer menstruating, your daily need decreases to 8 milligrams.

➤ **GOOD TO KNOW!** Most premenopausal women only get about 75 percent of the iron they need from food, so choosing iron-rich foods is especially important.

You read in chapter 7 about nutrient-packed produce such as pumpkin, which provides nearly three times your entire daily dose of vitamin A in just 1 cup, and Swiss chard, with six times your day's worth of vitamin K per cup. Now, in this chapter, you may notice that many of the Power Foods for healthy hair, nails, and teeth don't boast the same blockbuster proportions of Super Nutrients. The reason: most foods supply minerals in smaller doses, so you have to eat lots of mineral-rich foods to get your fill. So while it's easy to obtain more than an entire day's worth of vitamin C from 1 cup of papaya, you'd have to drink more than 3 cups of milk to get your day's calcium, or eat more than *2 pounds* of grilled sirloin steak for your entire day's iron. That's why I tell my clients it's just one more reason to focus on lots of different kinds of healthy whole foods.

➤ **SMART TIP** Calcium can block iron absorption. If you take a calcium supplement and a multivitamin containing iron, be sure to take them at different times of the day. It doesn't matter which you take first as long as you space them at least 3 hours apart.

➤ **DID YOU KNOW?** Spoon-shaped nails can be a sign of heart disease or an underactive thyroid, while other changes in your nails can reveal an underlying illness such as diabetes or a lung, liver, or kidney condition. If you notice something different about your nails' appearance, be sure to mention it to your doctor.

Where to Find It:
SIRLOIN STEAK

There's nothing like a juicy steak to help you get the iron you need for thick, strong hair and nails. But what about all that saturated fat? As it turns out, not all red meat is created equally where fat is concerned. Take sirloin steak—it's one of the leanest cuts of meat available, with just 4 grams of saturated fat and 11 grams of total fat per 4-ounce serving (the size of your palm). In return, it gives you 12 percent of your daily dose of readily absorbed heme iron (for more on heme iron, check out page 56 in chapter 4) with a moderate 240 calories.

➤ **GOOD TO KNOW!** Dark meat poultry, oysters, sardines, and tofu are also rich in iron.

➤ **SMART TIP** To make your steak more satisfying without upping portion size, pair it with mushrooms. Like steak, mushrooms have a beefy texture. Plus, they're rich in the savory flavor umami found in red meat.

➤ **DID YOU KNOW?** Other lean cuts of beef include eye of round, top round, bottom round, and flank steak.

➤ **BONUS!** Four ounces of broiled sirloin serve up three-quarters of your daily zinc, which you'll read about later in this chapter, as well as vitamin B_{12}, needed to help build keratin, a hair protein.

- ◆ Beef Stir-Fry, page 160
- ◆ Steak and Onion Tacos with Fresh Tomato Salsa, page 206

PHOSPHORUS

What It Is: This mineral is found in every single one of your cells. On the exterior, it's a vital part of the membranes that protect and line the cells. Inside, it helps manufacture proteins that cells need for growth and repair, and is a critical part of your DNA, ensuring that cells multiply properly. Phosphorus is also instrumental in converting food to fuel for energy, and, like calcium and potassium, maintaining your body's delicate acid-base balance.

How It Keeps Teeth Healthy: An impressive 85 percent of your body's phosphorus is found in your bones and teeth, where it teams up with calcium to keep them rock solid. And its benefits continue long after your teeth are fully formed. In fact, every time you

---

EAT SMART
How not to spoil your smile

Here are trouble-makers to avoid:

◆ **Anything sticky and sugary.** It doesn't matter if it's gooey caramel or vitamin-packed dried fruit, bacteria in your mouth love to feast on sticky carbs, wearing away tooth enamel and leading to tooth decay. Since it's not always practical to avoid sticky foods entirely, rinse your mouth with water afterward to wash away sugars that can encourage bacterial growth.

◆ **Soda and other drinks.** Sugar isn't the only reason soda spells trouble for your teeth. It also contains enamel-destroying acid. Meaning? Even if your soda is sugar-free, it can still do a number on your smile. Ditto for sports drinks and energy drinks, as both of these bathe your teeth in acid. Energy drinks are so harmful that a 2012 *General Dentistry* study found that they wear away twice as much protective enamel as sports drinks, because of the citric acid.

◆ **Chips.** Potato and tortilla chips might not seem like they're harmful to your smile, but little pieces of these carb-rich snacks can wedge themselves between teeth, providing food for bacteria in your mouth to thrive on.

◆ **Coffee and tea.** Otherwise healthy in moderation, these beverages can turn your teeth dark and dingy. When only a hot drink will do, chase yours down with a glass of water to rinse away any residue.

◆ **Alcohol.** It doesn't matter if it's a mojito or a martini, alcohol can dry your mouth, robbing you of acid-neutralizing saliva. When it comes to dry mouth, alcohol isn't the only culprit. Some medications, such as antidepressants and medication for high blood pressure, can have the same effect. In addition to drinking plenty of water, chewing sugarless gum can encourage saliva flow.

bite into a food that contains phosphorus, it helps safeguard and fortify your teeth from decay. Here's why: After a meal, bacteria in your mouth produce acid that can cause tiny, microscopic nicks in your teeth. When you eat phosphorus and calcium, they work like cement to fill in these tiny crevices before cavities have a chance to form.

➤ **FACT** You require 700 milligrams of phosphorus a day.

➤ **GOOD TO KNOW!** Phosphorus is the second most plentiful mineral in your body after calcium.

➤ **DID YOU KNOW?** Hormone replacement therapy (HRT) can lower your phosphorus levels by causing you to excrete more of this mineral. If you're on HRT, make sure to eat plenty of phosphorus-rich foods. In addition to the Power Foods in this chapter, you can find phosphorus in salmon, yogurt, milk, lean beef, poultry, and lentils.

Where to Find It:
WHEAT GERM
The embryo of the wheat kernel, wheat germ, is chock full of nutrients, including phosphorus. Sprinkle ¼ cup on your cereal or yogurt, and you'll rack up 46 percent of your day's phosphorus for a mere 108 calories. You'll also gain 4 grams of fiber to help keep you full—and scrub stains off your teeth.

➤ **QUICK IDEA** Next time you make chicken cutlets or bread fish fillets, swap in wheat germ for half of the breadcrumbs. Here's how: Dip boneless pieces in raw scrambled egg, then dip in the breadcrumb–wheat germ mixture, coating thoroughly on both sides. Spray a baking sheet with nonstick cooking spray. Transfer chicken or fish to baking sheet and bake in a 400°F oven for 25–30 minutes.

➤ **SMART TIP** Wheat germ contains small amounts of polyunsaturated fats. Even though these are healthy for your heart, they can cause wheat germ to go rancid quickly at room temperature. Store yours in the fridge for maximum freshness.

➤ **BONUS!** Wheat germ is jammed with other nutrients that keep you looking your best, such as vitamin E, iron, and zinc, which you'll read about later in this chapter.

RECIPE
◆ Raisin Spice Breakfast Sundae, page 143

PART-SKIM MOZZARELLA
Phosphorus- and calcium-packed dairy products, such as milk, yogurt, and cheese, are among the top foods for keeping your pearly whites in top shape. To see how different dairy products stack up against tooth decay, researchers in a 2013 *General Dentistry* study fed volunteers a snack of cheese, milk, yogurt, or a placebo. They then measured the amount of acid in volunteers' mouths. After 30 minutes, they found that milk and yogurt had stopped reducing acid, but the cheese was still going strong. In addition to acid-neutralizing phosphorus, researchers suspect cheese contains other components that encourage bacteria in your mouth to help lower acid.

➤ **QUICK IDEA** Instead of nibbling on cheese and crackers, sprinkle ¼ cup of shredded lowfat cheese on top of a sliced apple or pear and microwave for 30 seconds for a gooey fruit-and-cheese snack.

➤ **GOOD TO KNOW!** A quarter cup of part-skim shredded mozzarella contains only 4 grams of fat and 2.5 grams of saturated fat. Part-skim mozzarella string cheese is also a winner. These individually wrapped, single-serving cheese sticks make portion control a no-brainer with only 80 calories apiece.

➤ **BONUS!** A quarter cup of shredded part-skim mozzarella provides 5 grams of protein for only 65 calories.

RECIPES
♦ Broccoli and Tomato Pizza, page 150
♦ Cheesy Corn Tortillas, page 224
♦ Veggie Burger Parmesan, page 157

ZINC

What It Is: If there were an Academy Awards for nutrition, the Oscar for best supporting nutrient would go to zinc. This mineral assists in more than 100 different reactions in your body. At any given moment in time, it's helping you burn carbs, making proteins, detoxifying contaminants in your liver, and clearing away free radicals. If that weren't enough, it also assists your body in building DNA, boosts your immune system, encourages wounds to heal, and heightens your sense of smell and taste.

How It Keeps Hair and Nails Healthy:

Zinc is important for the formation of keratin, the protein that makes up hair and nails. So it's no surprise that a deficiency can make your hair shed and your nails chip.

➤ **FACT** You need 8 milligrams of zinc a day. Since your body can't store it, you need to eat it daily.

➤ **GOOD TO KNOW!** Between 35 and 45 percent of people over 60 don't get enough zinc.

➤ **SMART TIP** Plant foods like grains and beans are filled with substances called phytates, which hinder zinc absorption. If you're a vegetarian, you may need up to 50 percent more zinc than meat eaters.

➤ **DID YOU KNOW?** You lose zinc when you sweat, so if you workout strenuously or do hot yoga, it's especially important to eat a little extra on those days.

Where to Find It:
CLAMS

These shellfish contain all the minerals you need for healthy hair, nails, and teeth. In one appetizer of 10 small clams, you'll gain one-third of your daily dose of zinc, plus 46 and 15 percent, respectively, of your day's phosphorus and iron. Plus, you'll find 24 grams of lean protein — all for only 141 calories.

➤ **QUICK IDEAS** Don't feel you have to go out and buy a bucket of clams to steam yourself. Canned clams are a smart convenience food. Keep them on hand to toss into pasta marinara, sprinkle into paella, or use as a topping for pizza.

➤ **SMART TIP** If you're buying fresh clams, choose ones with shells that are closed. Open shells are a sign that clams are no longer fresh.

➤ **GOOD TO KNOW!** Beef, pork, poultry, yogurt, oysters, crab, cashews, and chickpeas are also rich in zinc.

➤ **DID YOU KNOW?** Farmed clams are low in mercury. In addition, they earn high marks for sustainability, as they're unlikely to disrupt other marine species, reports the Environmental Defense Fund.

➤ **BONUS!** Clams are an impressive source of hair-supporting vitamin B_{12}. Ten small

Mercury and hair loss

You may have heard that too much mercury in your diet can make your hair shed. That's because high levels of heavy metals in the blood, such as mercury, can be deposited in your hair follicles, where they can interfere with proper hair growth. While excessive mercury can technically cause hair loss, it might make you feel better to know that hair specialists rarely see this in real life. If it were to occur, you'd likely experience several other symptoms of mercury poisoning, such as memory loss, headaches, tremors, loss of coordination, and tingling in your hands and feet, too.

➤ **BOTTOM LINE:** While mercury can come from fish and shellfish, most of the mercury in seafood is concentrated in four species: shark, swordfish, tilefish, and king mackerel. As long as you avoid these four fish, it's safe to eat up to 12 ounces of seafood a week. One exception: if you're pregnant or plan to become pregnant, choose lower-mercury light canned tuna as well, and limit it to one can per week.

cooked clams contain 39 times the amount you require in a day.

RECIPE

+ Linguine with Tomatoes, Spinach, and Clams, page 182

OTHER POWER FOODS FOR HEALTHY HAIR AND NAILS

BONELESS CHICKEN BREASTS

How They Keep Hair and Nails Healthy: They're rich in protein.

If you're well nourished, you can expect to grow about ½ inch of new hair every month. Yet without enough protein, hair growth can slow. Dermatologists see this all the time when their patients are trying to slim down, detoxing, or have recently gone vegetarian or vegan. And even if you eat a balanced diet, it can be difficult to eat the protein you need throughout the day. That's where boneless chicken breasts come in. A 4-ounce grilled chicken breast gives you a hefty 35 grams of protein for a super-lean 171 calories.

➤ **SMART TIP** You can store raw chicken in the fridge for 2 days after you bring it home from the store. Cook it, and it keeps for 3 days.

➤ **FACT** If you're concerned about hormones in your chicken, you'll be glad to know that poultry farmers in the United States are not allowed to treat their birds with hormones.

➤ **GOOD TO KNOW!** After you marinate chicken, the leftover sauce is swimming in bacteria. If you like to drizzle a little extra marinade on your chicken after it's cooked, set some extra aside before you marinate to make sure it's bacteria-free.

RECIPES

+ Apple Spinach Salad, page 147
+ Asian Chicken Tacos, page 147

- Avocado Chicken, page 159
- Beet Tabbouleh with Grilled Chicken, page 162
- Cashew-Chicken Stir-Fry, page 164
- Chicken Vegetable Skewers, page 170
- Grilled Chicken Salad with Avocado and Grapefruit, page 178
- Kale Salad with Chicken and Cheddar, page 153
- Linguine with Chicken, Spinach, and Mushrooms, page 182
- Walnut-Crusted Chicken Cutlets, page 209

FENNEL

How It Keeps Teeth Healthy: It's rich in fiber.

Fibrous fennel is like nature's toothbrush, scrubbing stains from your teeth so they stay whiter and brighter. Since fennel requires lots of chewing, it also stimulates acid-neutralizing saliva. Toss 1 cup of fennel slices into a salad (or munch on it as a snack), and you'll net close to 3 grams of roughage for only 27 calories.

➤ QUICK IDEAS Fennel has a licorice flavor, so it also makes a tasty swap for celery in crudités. And don't toss the fronds—finely chop them and sprinkle over a sautéed filet of sole, or some shrimp, with a squeeze of lemon juice.

➤ GOOD TO KNOW! Fennel is great for your gums, too. One cup serves up 14 percent of your daily vitamin C, a nutrient that keeps gums healthy so they don't become red and puffy.

➤ BONUS! Fennel is loaded with bone-building vitamin K. One cup provides 61 percent of your daily requirement.

➤ DID YOU KNOW? Strawberries are another natural smile-whitener, thanks to tiny seeds that scour away stains.

RECIPE
- Corkscrew Pasta with Sausage and Fennel, page 172

GREEN BEANS

How They Keep Hair and Nails Healthy: They're rich in silicon.

Like biotin, which you'll read more about on page 130, silicon helps chip-proof nails. When women in a Belgian study downed a daily supplement containing 10 milligrams of silicon for 5 months, their nails became significantly less brittle than women in a control group who popped a placebo. Studies show that silicon may also reduce signs of aging by strengthening hair and diminishing skin wrinkles. Silicon, however, can be tricky to find in foods. Even though it's in produce like bananas and carrots, it's not always well absorbed. Green beans deliver one of the most easily utilized forms of silicon—as do raisins, bran flakes, and—surprise—beer.

➤ GOOD TO KNOW! Health experts recommend that you consume 5–20 milligrams of silicon a day, though there is no established requirement.

➤ SMART TIP Green beans have a surprisingly long shelf life. Store them in a plastic bag in your fridge, and they'll stay fresh for up to 5 days.

➤ DID YOU KNOW? They are also a skin-friendly food, thanks to plenty of vitamin C.

➤ BONUS! A cup of cooked green beans gives you nearly 4 grams of fiber.

RECIPE
- Slow Cooker Italian Lentil and Vegetable Stew, page 199

HERRING

How It Keeps Hair Healthy: It's rich in protein.

When you hardly have time to cook, getting the protein you need can be a challenge. Why not give herring a try? You can find it ready-made—either plain, pickled, or in wine sauce. All you have to do is pop open the jar! Two ounces of this convenient fish (about ¼ cup) give you as much protein as in one egg.

➤ QUICK IDEAS Try herring Scandinavian-style with a slice of pumpernickel for breakfast, or on a rye crisp with mustard for a speedy snack.

➤ GOOD TO KNOW! Herring is in season in the springtime. If you'd like to try it but you're not inclined to cook it, order it in your favorite fish restaurant.

➤ BONUS! Fish is an outstanding source of enamel-building phosphorus. Four ounces of fresh herring gives you 38 percent of your daily dose. It also serves up six times your recommended vitamin B_{12}.

RECIPE

◆ Open-Faced Pickled Herring Sandwich, page 154

OATS

How They Keep Nails Healthy: They're rich in biotin.

Experts first suspected this nutrient might improve nail health after learning that horses whose feed contained extra biotin had hooves that were less brittle and prone to splitting. Now, they're finding this vitamin may help humans, too. In a Swiss study, people with brittle nails who downed 2,500 micrograms of supplemental biotin every day for 6–15 months grew nails that were 25 percent thicker. Their

---

ALL ABOARD!
Entice your family to eat more fish

If your clan won't bite, try these no-fail tricks:

1 **Mix it with an old favorite.** Help your family warm up to seafood by pairing it with something they already love. Try shrimp over linguine marinara, tilapia tacos, or tuna sliders.

2 **Cut down on the smell factor.** Fish isn't always the best-smelling food. Baking it instead of pan-frying it can go a long way in keeping fishy odors from hijacking your kitchen. The recipe for Greek-Style Tilapia on page 175 makes it simple.

3 **Infuse it with flavor.** Make salmon or tuna steaks even tastier by marinating them before cooking (check out "Marinate It!" on page 59 in chapter 4 for suggestions).

4 **Let them eat cake.** If fish fillets are a no-go in your house, try crab or salmon cakes (such as the Salmon Cakes recipe on page 194). Their burger-like shape and texture makes them much friendlier to seafood novices.

5 **Pick a winner.** Even people who usually turn up their nose at fish will eat shrimp cocktail. Buy it precooked from the grocery store, and serve it with a big salad and some crusty bread for a dinner that's ready in 5 minutes flat.

nails were also smoother and less likely to split. However, the 2,500–3,000 daily micrograms of biotin that dermatologists recommend for stronger nails is considerably more than you could ever get from food alone. So if you're striving for that much, you'll need a supplement (if that sounds like a lot, biotin is considered to be extremely safe in these amounts). If you'd prefer a natural biotin boost, start your morning with a bowl of oatmeal. One half cup of uncooked oats boasts 30 percent of the 30 micrograms of biotin you need each day.

➤ **SMART TIP** You'll likely need to take or eat extra biotin for several months before you see the results. And even though it can strengthen brittle nails, it won't make healthy nails thicker.

➤ **QUICK IDEA** Swap oats in for breadcrumbs in meatloaf or meatballs for more nail-friendly biotin plus added fiber.

➤ **BONUS!** Oats are a top source of beta-glucan, a special kind of fiber that lowers cholesterol, as well as avenanthramides, powerful antioxidants that keep your arteries clear of plaque.

➤ **DID YOU KNOW?** In addition to oats, you can find biotin in pecans, egg yolks, beans, cauliflower, bananas, mushrooms, and sardines.

RECIPES
- Maple Almond Oatmeal, page 141
- PB & Banana Oatmeal, page 142

TILAPIA
How It Keeps Hair Healthy: It's rich in vitamin D.

If your tresses are starting to thin, you may want to make sure you're consuming enough vitamin D. When researchers in a 2013 *Skin Pharmacology and Physiology* study measured levels of this vitamin in women with chronic hair loss, they found that the less vitamin D the women had in their blood, the sparser their hair was. One reason may be vitamin D's role in regulating hair's life cycle. Normally, hair goes through three different phases: a growth stage, a brief period when growth slows, and a final phase when hair stops growing and eventually falls out. Once the cycle is complete, it usually starts anew. But recent research reveals that if you're not getting enough vitamin D, hair may not grow back again after it falls out, resulting in fewer strands overall. Mild-tasting tilapia is an easy way to work more D into your diet. One 4-ounce filet gives you a roughly a quarter of your daily requirement. To learn other ways to add vitamin D to your diet, check out "Eat Smart: Get the Vitamin D You Need" on page 94 in chapter 6.

➤ **SMART TIP** For the most sustainably raised tilapia, choose tank-farmed fillets from the United States or Canada.

➤ **QUICK IDEA** When you need a good-for-you meal in a hurry, try this: season a tilapia fillet with garlic powder, sea salt, pepper, and lemon zest, and bake on a baking sheet sprayed with nonstick cooking spray in a 375°F oven for 25–30 minutes.

➤ **BONUS!** Tilapia is packed with lean protein. Four ounces deliver 30 grams for only 145 calories and less than 3 grams of fat.

RECIPE
- Greek-Style Tilapia, page 175

One-week meal plan for healthier hair, nails, and teeth

	BREAKFAST	LUNCH	DINNER
DAY 1	Maple Almond Oatmeal*	Veggie Burger Parmesan* 1 apple	Greek-Style Tilapia* 1 cup cooked peas with 1 teaspoon olive oil
DAY 2	Raisin Spice Breakfast Sundae*	BBQ Turkey Burger* 1 cup grape tomatoes	Corkscrew Pasta with Sausage and Fennel*
DAY 3	Huevos Rancheros*	Open-Faced Pickled Herring Sandwich* 3/4 cup grapes	Chicken Vegetable Skewers* Roasted Pears*
DAY 4	Cantaloupe Breakfast Bowl*	Broccoli and Tomato Pizza*	Spiced Pork Tenderloins with Mango Salsa* 1/4 cup quinoa, cooked according to package directions 1 cup green beans drizzled with 2 teaspoons olive oil
DAY 5	Apricot Ricotta Breakfast Sundae*	Curried Chickpea Pita*	Linguine with Tomatoes, Spinach, and Clams*
DAY 6	1 cup toasted oat cereal 2 tablespoons toasted wheat germ 1/2 sliced banana 1 cup 1% milk	Tuna Cheddar Melt* 3/4 cup pineapple chunks	Slow Cooker Italian Lentil and Vegetable Stew* 1/2 cup sliced strawberries mixed with 1/2 cup pomegranate seeds
DAY 7	Sunrise Smoothie* (if desired, substitute 2 tablespoons toasted wheat germ for 1 tablespoon chia seeds)	Kale Salad with Chicken and Cheddar*	Beef Stir-Fry* 1 cup asparagus sautéed in 1 teaspoon canola oil

*Recipe included in chapter 9

1 piece part-skim mozzarella string cheese + ¾ cup grapes

1 hardboiled egg sprinkled with curry powder + 8 small whole-grain crackers

6 ounces nonfat plain Greek yogurt with ½ cup sliced strawberries and 1 tablespoon wheat germ

PB and Banana "Sandwich"*

15 pecan halves

1 apple and 2 1-inch Brie cubes

Chia Pudding*

1 celery stalk filled with 1 ½ tablespoons almond butter

Cheesy Corn Tortillas*

¾ cup edamame

Ambrosia Parfaits*

1 cup sliced fennel dipped in ¼ cup hummus

1 cup sliced red and yellow peppers dipped in ¼ cup guacamole

¼ cup part-skim ricotta mixed with 1 teaspoon fresh herbs (such as parsley or tarragon) on 8 small whole-wheat crackers

CHECKLIST
For better hair, nails, and teeth

○ A diet rich in minerals is essential for stronger hair, nails, and teeth. Get yours from a balanced diet that contains plenty of whole foods.

○ If your nails are brittle, eat biotin-rich foods like oats and consider a biotin supplement. You can also protect nails by wearing rubber gloves when you wash dishes and avoiding harsh detergents.

○ For healthy snacking, nibble on tooth-supporting dairy products, like lowfat cheese or yogurt, as well as fibrous foods, like fennel or celery.

○ To improve hair and nails, don't forget to eat zinc-rich foods every day, such as clams, lean cuts of beef and pork, poultry, nuts, yogurt, and chickpeas.

○ Toss sliced or diced chicken breast into main dish salads and pasta, couscous, quinoa, and rice for extra lean protein.

○ For extra vitamin D, eat more seafood by serving at least two fish meals a week. Top sources include tilapia, salmon, and sardines.

○ If you drink coffee or tea, sip some water or rinse your mouth afterward to wash away residue that can stain your teeth. Ditto for sticky or sweet foods.

○ And to ease a dry mouth, water and sugarless gum can help.

CHAPTER 9

Delicious Anti-Aging Recipes and Meal Plans

Every single recipe in this chapter contains at least one (and sometimes several) of the anti-aging Power Foods you've read about in earlier chapters. Your mission: try as many as possible!

Gooey Strawberry French Toast, Mediterranean Steak Salad, Slow Cooker Butternut Squash Barley Risotto, and Good-for-You Hot Chocolate—these are just some of the 96 tasty recipes that will put this book's promise into practice: helping you stay healthy, have more energy, and look your best. And the nutrition-packed meals are surprisingly slimming. Each day, you'll eat about 300 calories for breakfast, 400 at lunch, and 500 for dinner. You're also free to indulge in at least two 150-calorie snacks to fill every craving, from sweet, to salty, to savory, to crunchy. Had a big workout one day and need more calories than the 1,500-calorie guide offers? Simply add a snack. Need fewer calories? Subtract a snack. Men can have three snacks, or if they're highly active, two snacks that are double in size.

To get you in and out of the kitchen quickly, breakfast, lunch, and snacks involve no more than 10–15 minutes to pull together. Plus, they're conveniently sized for one person. If you're cooking for two or more, just double, triple, or quadruple the ingredients. Since evening is the perfect time to sit down over a good meal with family or friends, dinner is a little different. Dishes are designed to feed four people, and recipes take only 35–45 minutes to finish (and plenty require only 15 minutes or less!). The handful of exceptions are short-prep recipes that require a little more cooking time, such as Slow Cooker Chicken Marbella on page 198 or the baked Ziti with Eggplant and Ricotta on page 210.

At the end of this chapter, you'll find four meal plans. The first is a master meal plan packed with recipes that tackle every angle of anti-aging eating, from reducing your risk for many diseases, to diminishing wrinkles, to boosting your brainpower. Alternately, if you're on a special diet—gluten-free, low-carb, or vegetarian—there's a special meal plan designed just for you.

So what are you waiting for? It's time to start cooking!

KEY FOR SPECIAL DIETS
GF Gluten-free
LC Low-carb
V Vegetarian

NEW WAYS TO SEASON TO TASTE

In many of the recipes in this chapter you'll see the words "**season to taste**." Adding a little seasoning to your meals isn't limited to salt and pepper. It can alternatively be a squeeze of lemon or lime juice, a sprinkle of fresh or dried herbs, or a few shakes of garlic or chili powder. If you do choose to add salt, use no more than a pinch per serving. Every extra pinch contributes an additional 300 milligrams of sodium to each recipe, over and above the amount listed in the nutrition stats.

BREAKFAST

APRICOT RICOTTA BREAKFAST SUNDAE

MAKES 1 serving

GOOD FOR:
Strength, skin, hair, nails, and teeth

Whisk **¾ cup part-skim ricotta** with **½ teaspoon honey** and **1 pinch nutmeg**. Top with **two chopped apricots (either fresh or dried)**.

EACH SERVING ABOUT: *309 calories, 21 g protein, 20 g carbohydrate, 15 g total fat (9 g saturated fat), 233 mg sodium, 520 mg calcium, 1 g fiber, 130 mg omega-3*

AVOCADO SWISS BREAKFAST SANDWICH

MAKES 1 serving

GOOD FOR: *Blood sugar, brain, strength, hair, nails, and teeth*

Toast **1 whole-wheat English muffin**. Divide in half. Spread each half with **1 teaspoon Dijon mustard**. Top one half with **1 slice Swiss cheese, ¼ sliced avocado,** and **1 slice tomato**. Season to taste. Cover with remaining English muffin half.

EACH SERVING ABOUT: *307 calories, 14 g protein, 33 g carbohydrate, 15 g total fat (6 g saturated fat), 537 mg sodium, 268 mg calcium, 7 g fiber, 140 mg omega-3*

BETTER-FOR-YOU BLUEBERRY WAFFLES

MAKES 1 serving

GOOD FOR: *Heart, blood sugar, cancer prevention, brain, strength, skin, hair, nails, and teeth*

Whisk **¼ cup part-skim ricotta cheese** with **1 large pinch cinnamon**. Divide in half and spread over **2 toasted whole-grain waffles**. Top each waffle with **¼ cup blueberries**.

EACH SERVING ABOUT: *309 calories, 13 g protein, 42 g carbohydrate, 11 g total fat (4 g saturated fat), 498 mg sodium, 276 mg calcium, 5 g fiber, 90 mg omega-3*

GOOD FOR: *Heart, blood sugar, cancer prevention, brain, strength, skin, hair, nails, and teeth*

BREAKFAST BURRITO

MAKES 1 serving

In a medium sauté pan, cook **1 scrambled egg** in **1 teaspoon canola oil**. Season to taste. Transfer egg to a warmed **8-inch whole-wheat tortilla**. Top tortilla with **¼ cup warmed rinsed and drained no-salt-added canned black beans, ¼ cup diced tomato, ¼ red or yellow bell pepper (chopped)**, and **1 tablespoon chopped sweet onion**.

EACH SERVING ABOUT: *316 calories, 14 g protein, 38 g carbohydrate, 13 g total fat (3 g saturated fat), 396 mg sodium, 62 mg calcium, 7 g fiber, 430 mg omega-3*

GF V

GOOD FOR: *Heart, blood sugar, cancer prevention, brain, strength, skin, hair, nails, and teeth*

CANTALOUPE BREAKFAST BOWL

MAKES 1 serving

Fold **½ cup blueberries** and **1 pinch cinnamon** into **⅓ cup part-skim ricotta cheese**. Spoon mixture into **½ hollowed-out cantaloupe**. Top with **1 tablespoon sliced almonds**.

EACH SERVING ABOUT: *290 calories, 13 g protein, 40 g carbohydrate, 10 g total fat (4 g saturated fat), 144 mg sodium, 286 mg calcium, 5 g fiber, 100 mg omega-3*

CREAMY ORANGE BANANA WAFFLE

MAKES 1 serving

GOOD FOR: *Brain, strength, hair, nails, and teeth*

Spread **2 teaspoons orange marmalade** on **1 toasted whole-grain waffle**. Top with **½ cup 1% cottage cheese** and **1 sliced banana**.

EACH SERVING ABOUT: *309 calories, 18 g protein, 53 g carbohydrate, 5 g total fat (1 g saturated fat), 677 mg sodium, 130 mg calcium, 5 g fiber, 40 mg omega-3*

CRUNCHY SUNFLOWER BUTTER SANDWICH

MAKES 1 serving

GOOD FOR: *Heart, blood sugar, cancer prevention, brain, skin, hair, nails, and teeth*

Cut **an apple** in half and cut into slices, removing core. Spread **1 tablespoon sunflower butter** on **1 slice whole-wheat toast**. Top with **1 tablespoon sunflower seeds** and **½ sliced apple**. Serve with remaining sliced apple.

EACH SERVING ABOUT: *287 calories, 7 g protein, 41 g carbohydrate, 13 g total fat (1 g saturated fat), 213 mg sodium, 18 mg calcium, 9 g fiber, 10 mg omega-3*

(V)

GOOD FOR: *Cancer prevention, brain, strength, and skin*

GOOEY STRAWBERRY FRENCH TOAST

MAKES 1 serving

In a microwave oven, heat **1 cup frozen strawberries, 1 teaspoon sugar**, and **¼ teaspoon orange zest** for 1 minute, or until just warmed. Set aside. In a shallow bowl, whisk **1 egg**. Dip **1 slice whole-wheat bread** into egg. In a medium sauté pan, fry bread in **1 teaspoon butter** until golden brown, about 4 minutes, flipping halfway. Serve **strawberries** over French toast.

EACH SERVING ABOUT: *266 calories, 12 g protein, 37 g carbohydrate, 9 g total fat (4 g saturated fat), 181 mg sodium, 82 mg calcium, 6 g fiber, 10 mg omega-3*

GOOD FOR: *Blood sugar, cancer prevention, strength, hair, nails, and teeth*

HUEVOS RANCHEROS

MAKES 1 serving

In a medium sauté pan, cook **1 scrambled egg** in **1 teaspoon canola oil**. Season to taste. Transfer egg to a warmed **6-inch corn tortilla**. Top tortilla with **½ cup warmed rinsed and drained no-salt-added canned black beans, ¼ cup nonfat plain Greek yogurt**, and **2 tablespoons salsa**.

EACH SERVING ABOUT: *304 calories, 19 g protein, 34 g carbohydrate, 10 g total fat (2 g saturated fat), 334 mg sodium, 118 mg calcium, 8 g fiber, 430 mg omega-3*

MAPLE ALMOND OATMEAL

MAKES 1 serving

GOOD FOR: *Heart, cancer prevention, brain, strength, skin, hair, nails, and teeth*

Prepare **½ cup oats** according to package directions. Swirl in **1 tablespoon almond butter**. Top with **½ cup 1% milk** and drizzle with **1 teaspoon 100% pure maple syrup**.

EACH SERVING ABOUT: *317 calories, 12 g protein, 41 g carbohydrate, 13 g total fat (2 g saturated fat), 91 mg sodium, 215 mg calcium, 6 g fiber, 10 mg omega-3*

ORANGE AND APRICOT QUINOA

MAKES 1 serving

GOOD FOR: *Heart, cancer prevention, brain, and skin*

In a medium saucepan, prepare **¼ cup quinoa** according to package directions, substituting **orange juice** for half of the water and adding **1 large pinch cinnamon**. Once quinoa is cooked, uncover, fluff with fork, and stir in **four chopped dried apricots** and **1 tablespoon sliced almonds**.

EACH SERVING ABOUT: *300 calories, 8 g protein, 55 g carbohydrate, 6 g total fat (1 g saturated fat), 6 mg sodium, 143 mg calcium, 7 g fiber, 140 mg omega-3*

GOOD FOR: *Heart,*
cancer prevention,
brain, hair, nails,
and teeth

PB & BANANA OATMEAL

MAKES 1 serving

Prepare **½ cup oats** according to package directions. Stir in
1 tablespoon peanut butter. Top with **½ sliced banana** and
1 teaspoon 100% pure maple syrup.

EACH SERVING ABOUT: *314 calories, 9 g protein, 49 g carbohydrate,*
11 g total fat (2 g saturated fat), 78 mg sodium, 18 mg calcium, 6 g fiber,
20 mg omega-3

GOOD FOR: *Heart,*
cancer prevention,
brain, strength,
hair, nails, and
teeth

PEACH BLUEBERRY SMOOTHIE

MAKES 1 serving

In a blender, purée **1 cup lowfat plain kefir** with **1 cup frozen
peaches**, **1 cup frozen blueberries**, **1 teaspoon honey**,
1 tablespoon ground flaxseed, and **a pinch of nutmeg**
until smooth.

EACH SERVING ABOUT: *293 calories, 14 g protein, 53 g carbohydrate,*
5 g total fat (2 g saturated fat), 127 mg sodium, 323 mg calcium, 8 g fiber,
1,370 mg omega-3

POMEGRANATE-APRICOT BREAKFAST CROSTINI

MAKES 1 serving

In a small bowl, whisk **2 teaspoons apricot jam** into **¼ cup part-skim ricotta cheese**. Divide and spread over **1 toasted whole-wheat English muffin**. Sprinkle with **1 tablespoon pomegranate seeds** and **1 tablespoon sunflower seeds**.

EACH SERVING ABOUT: *304 calories, 15 g protein, 42 g carbohydrate, 10 g total fat (4 g saturated fat), 325 mg sodium, 358 mg calcium, 6 g fiber, 70 mg omega-3*

GOOD FOR: *Heart, cancer prevention, brain, strength, skin, hair, nails, and teeth*

RAISIN SPICE BREAKFAST SUNDAE

MAKES 1 serving

In a small bowl, whisk **1 cup nonfat plain yogurt** with **1 teaspoon honey** and **1 pinch each nutmeg and cinnamon**. Top with **1 tablespoon raisins, 1 tablespoon wheat germ,** and **1 tablespoon chopped pecans**.

EACH SERVING ABOUT: *290 calories, 16 g protein, 36 g carbohydrate, 10 g total fat (3 g saturated fat), 175 mg sodium, 466 mg calcium, 2 g fiber, 100 mg omega-3*

GOOD FOR: *Heart, brain, strength, hair, nails, and teeth*

GOOD FOR: *Heart, blood sugar, cancer prevention, brain, strength, skin, hair, nails, and teeth*

MAKE IT A MEAL!
Serve with
1 medium orange.

SPINACH-FETA OMELET

MAKES 1 serving

In a medium bowl, scramble **1 egg** with **3 egg whites**. Heat **1 teaspoon olive oil** in a medium sauté pan over medium-low heat. Add egg. Stir in **1 cup chopped baby spinach** and **1 tablespoon crumbled feta cheese** and cook until eggs are firm. Season to taste. Fold and serve.

EACH SERVING ABOUT: *194 calories, 19 g protein, 5 g carbohydrate, 11 g total fat (3 g saturated fat), 323 mg sodium, 69 mg calcium, 1 g fiber, 0 mg omega-3*

GOOD FOR: *Heart, cancer prevention, brain, strength, skin, hair, nails, and teeth*

SUNRISE SMOOTHIE

MAKES 1 serving

In a blender, purée **1 cup papaya cubes** with **½ frozen banana**, **½ cup orange juice**, **½ cup nonfat plain Greek yogurt**, and **1 tablespoon chia seeds** until smooth.

EACH SERVING ABOUT: *287 calories, 16 g protein, 50 g carbohydrate, 5 g total fat (1 g saturated fat), 56 mg sodium, 234 mg calcium, 8 g fiber, 1,970 mg omega-3*

TROPICAL GREEK YOGURT BREAKFAST PARFAIT

MAKES 1 serving

GOOD FOR: *Heart, blood sugar, cancer prevention, brain, strength, skin, hair, nails, and teeth*

In a blender combine **6 ounces nonfat plain Greek yogurt** with **½ sliced banana** and purée until smooth. Spoon half of banana-yogurt mixture into a bowl or parfait glass. Top with **½ cup drained pineapple chunks in water**. Spoon remaining banana-yogurt mixture over pineapple. Top with **2 tablespoons sliced toasted almonds** and **2 teaspoons shredded unsweetened coconut**.

EACH SERVING ABOUT: *309 calories, 23 g protein, 35 g carbohydrate, 10 g total fat (3 g saturated fat), 83 mg sodium, 262 mg calcium, 5 g fiber, 30 mg omega-3*

LUNCH

APPLE SPINACH SALAD

MAKES 1 serving

GF

GOOD FOR: *Heart, blood sugar, cancer prevention, strength, skin, hair, nails, and teeth*

In a medium bowl, toss **3 cups baby spinach** with **1 diced apple**, **½ cup grated carrots**, **½ cup shredded skinless rotisserie chicken breast**, **1 tablespoon olive oil**, and **1 tablespoon balsamic vinegar**. Season to taste. Top with **1 tablespoon pumpkin seeds**.

EACH SERVING ABOUT: *406 calories, 25 g protein, 40 g carbohydrate, 17 g total fat (3 g saturated fat), 210 mg sodium, 87 mg calcium, 11 g fiber, 150 mg omega-3*

ASIAN CHICKEN TACOS

MAKES 1 serving

LC

GOOD FOR: *Heart, blood sugar, cancer prevention, brain, strength, hair, nails, and teeth*

GLUTEN-FREE VERSION: *Omit soy sauce and substitute **a gluten-free tamari sauce**.*

In a medium bowl, combine **⅔ cup shredded skinless rotisserie chicken breast**, **1 cup baby spinach**, **1 tablespoon chopped peanuts**, and **½ sliced scallion**. Drizzle with **1½ teaspoons peanut oil**, **1½ teaspoons reduced-sodium soy sauce**, and **1½ teaspoons rice wine vinegar**, and toss. Season to taste. Warm **2 6-inch corn tortillas** on a griddle or in a large sauté pan for 1 minute. Top each tortilla with half of taco mixture.

EACH SERVING ABOUT: *395 calories, 35 g protein, 27 g carbohydrate, 17 g total fat (3 g saturated fat), 402 mg sodium, 42 mg calcium, 4 g fiber, 70 mg omega-3*

BAKED POTATO "BURRITO BOWL"

MAKES 1 serving

Split **1 medium baked potato** in half. Scoop out flesh with a spoon and mash with **3 tablespoons reduced-fat shredded cheddar cheese** and **¼ cup nonfat plain Greek yogurt**. Season to taste. Divide in half. Stuff each potato skin half with half of the potato mixture. In a small bowl, toss **½ cup warmed rinsed and drained no-salt-added canned pinto beans** with **¼ cup microwaved frozen corn**, **1 sliced scallion**, **¼ cup diced tomato**, and **1 tablespoon fresh lime juice**. Divide in half and spoon over potatoes. Top each potato half with **2 tablespoons nonfat plain Greek yogurt**.

EACH SERVING ABOUT: *404 calories, 27 g protein, 70 g carbohydrate, 2 g total fat (1 g saturated fat), 211 mg sodium, 266 mg calcium, 12 g fiber, 40 mg omega-3*

BARLEY-STUFFED PEPPER

MAKES 1 serving

Prepare **¼ cup barley** according to package directions. In a medium bowl, toss cooked barley with **1 tablespoon crumbled feta cheese**, **⅓ cup microwaved frozen corn**, and **2 tablespoons chopped sweet onion** that's been sautéed in **1 teaspoon olive oil**. Season to taste. Stuff into **one hollowed red bell pepper**.

EACH SERVING ABOUT: *328 calories, 9 g protein, 59 g carbohydrate, 8 g total fat (2 g saturated fat), 66 mg sodium, 54 mg calcium, 12 g fiber, 60 mg omega-3*

BBQ TURKEY BURGER

MAKES 1 serving

Grill or broil a **4-ounce ground turkey breast patty**. Serve on **a toasted whole-wheat hamburger bun** with **1 slice Cheddar cheese**, **1 slice onion**, **2 slices of tomato**, and **1 tablespoon barbeque sauce**.

EACH SERVING ABOUT: *402 calories, 32 g protein, 33 g carbohydrate, 17 g total fat (7 g saturated fat), 608 mg sodium, 208 mg calcium, 4 g fiber, 50 mg omega-3*

LC

GOOD FOR: *Blood sugar, brain, strength, hair, nails, and teeth*

MAKE IT A MEAL! *Serve with* **remaining tomato**, *sliced. Season to taste.*

BLACK BEAN BURGER SALAD

MAKES 1 serving

In a small bowl, whisk **2 tablespoons fresh lime juice** with **1 tablespoon canola oil** and **1 pinch chili powder**. Drizzle over **2 cups shredded romaine lettuce**, **1/2 cup diced tomato**, **1/4 cup chopped sweet onion**, and **1/4 diced avocado**. Season to taste. Top with **1 cooked black bean burger patty**. Serve with **7 blue corn tortilla chips**.

EACH SERVING ABOUT: *398 calories, 9 g protein, 40 g carbohydrate, 26 g total fat (2 g saturated fat), 437 mg sodium, 102 mg calcium, 12 g fiber, 1,440 mg omega-3*

V

GOOD FOR: *Heart, blood sugar, cancer prevention, brain, and skin*

BLACK BEAN TOMATO SOUP

MAKES 1 serving

(V)

GOOD FOR: *Cancer prevention, brain, strength, skin, hair, nails, and teeth*

Mix **1¼ cups reduced-sodium tomato soup** with **2 teaspoons red wine vinegar**, **¾ cup rinsed and drained no-salt-added canned black beans**, **½ cup microwaved frozen corn**, **½ red or yellow bell pepper (chopped)**, **½ cup chopped tomato**, and **2 tablespoons chopped red onion**. Season to taste. Chill for 30 minutes before serving.

EACH SERVING ABOUT: 383 calories, 20 g protein, 71 g carbohydrate, 3 g total fat (2 g saturated fat), 707 mg sodium, 298 mg calcium, 15 g fiber, 20 mg omega-3

BROCCOLI AND TOMATO PIZZA

MAKES 1 serving

(V)

GOOD FOR: *Cancer prevention, brain, strength, skin, hair, nails, and teeth*

In a medium skillet, heat **1 teaspoon olive oil** over medium heat. Add **½ teaspoon minced garlic** and sauté for minute. Add **½ cup steamed broccoli**. Toss well and set aside.

Place a **6½ inch whole-wheat pita** on a baking sheet. Spread **2 tablespoons marinara sauce** over pita. Top with broccoli mixture, **¼ cup quartered grape tomatoes**, and **¼ cup part-skim ricotta cheese**. Sprinkle with **2 tablespoons part-skim shredded mozzarella**. Bake in a 475°F oven for 8–10 minutes.

EACH SERVING ABOUT: 381 calories, 21 g protein, 48 g carbohydrate, 15 g total fat (5 g saturated fat), 680 mg sodium, 432 mg calcium, 8 g fiber, 180 mg omega-3

BROWN RICE EDAMAME SALAD

MAKES 1 serving

Prepare **¼ cup brown rice** according to package directions. Toss with **½ cup microwaved frozen shelled edamame**, **¼ cup grated carrots**, **1 sliced scallion**, **1 teaspoon canola oil**, **2 teaspoons rice wine vinegar**, **2 teaspoons reduced-sodium soy sauce**. Season to taste. Sprinkle with **2 tablespoons sesame seeds**.

EACH SERVING ABOUT: *402 calories, 15 g protein, 48 g carbohydrate, 17 g total fat (1 g saturated fat), 444 mg sodium, 129 mg calcium, 7 g fiber, 450 mg omega-3*

GOOD FOR: *Heart, blood sugar, cancer prevention, brain, strength, skin, hair, nails, and teeth*

GLUTEN-FREE VERSION: *Omit soy sauce and substitute* **a gluten-free tamari sauce.**

COUSCOUS WITH CHICKPEAS

MAKES 1 serving

In a medium bowl, combine **1½ teaspoons extra virgin olive oil**, **¼ teaspoon lemon zest**, **1 tablespoon chopped fresh basil**, **¼ diced cucumber**, **½ cup chopped tomatoes**, and **½ cup warmed rinsed and drained no-salt-added canned chickpeas**. Add **¼ cup whole-wheat couscous** that has been prepared according to package directions. Season to taste. Toss well to combine.

EACH SERVING ABOUT: *391 calories, 16 g protein, 66 g carbohydrate, 9 g total fat (1 g saturated fat), 35 mg sodium, 100 mg calcium, 13 g fiber, 60 mg omega-3*

GOOD FOR: *Heart, blood sugar, cancer prevention, brain, strength, skin, hair, nails, and teeth*

GLUTEN-FREE VERSION: *Swap in* **¼ cup quinoa** *for whole-wheat couscous.*

GOOD FOR: *Heart, blood sugar, cancer prevention, brain, strength, skin, hair, nails, and teeth*

CURRIED CHICKPEA PITA

MAKES 1 serving

In a medium bowl, toss together **⅓ cup rinsed and drained no-salt-added canned chickpeas, 1 tablespoon raisins, ¼ cup grated carrots, 2 teaspoons fresh lime juice, 1 teaspoon extra virgin olive oil**, and **¼ teaspoon curry powder**. Season to taste. Stuff mixture into a **6½-inch whole-wheat pita**. Top with **¼ cup nonfat plain Greek yogurt**.

EACH SERVING ABOUT: *377 calories, 17 g protein, 64 g carbohydrate, 7 g total fat (1 g saturated fat), 347 mg sodium, 99 mg calcium, 10 g fiber, 70 mg omega-3*

GOOD FOR: *Blood sugar, cancer prevention, brain, strength, skin, hair, nails, and teeth*

MAKE IT A MEAL! *Serve with **12 multigrain pita chips***.

GRILLED SHRIMP CAESAR

MAKES 1 serving

Toss **3 cups chopped romaine lettuce** with **10 large grilled or boiled peeled shrimp** and **2 tablespoons Caesar dressing**. Season to taste. Top with **1 tablespoon grated Parmesan cheese**.

EACH SERVING ABOUT: *270 calories, 17 g protein, 7 g carbohydrate, 20 g total fat (4 g saturated fat), 964 mg sodium, 166 mg calcium, 3 g fiber, 1,470 mg omega-3*

KALE SALAD
WITH CHICKEN AND CHEDDAR

MAKES 1 serving

In a medium bowl, whisk together **1½ teaspoons lemon juice**, **1½ teaspoons extra virgin olive oil**, **1 teaspoon Worcestershire sauce**, **1½ teaspoons cider vinegar**, **½ teaspoon sugar**, and **1 pinch each kosher salt and ground black pepper**. Add **2 cups shredded kale**, **1 tablespoon dried tart cherries**, **1 tablespoon pine nuts**, **½ cup skinless shredded rotisserie chicken breast**, and **2 tablespoons reduced-fat shredded cheddar cheese**. Toss well.

EACH SERVING ABOUT: *379 calories, 33 g protein, 24 g carbohydrate, 19 g total fat (4 g saturated fat), 484 mg sodium, 325 mg calcium, 5 g fiber, 350 mg omega-3*

LC

GOOD FOR: *Blood sugar, cancer prevention, brain, strength, skin, hair, nails, and teeth*

GLUTEN-FREE VERSION: *Omit Worcestershire sauce or choose* **a gluten-free Worcestershire sauce**.

MEDITERRANEAN PASTA SALAD

MAKES 1 serving

Prepare **1 ounce dried whole-wheat pasta** according to package directions. Drain and toss with **½ cup rinsed and drained no-salt-added canned chickpeas**, **5 halved grape tomatoes**, **1 cup baby spinach**, **¼ cup part-skim shredded mozzarella**, **2 chopped fresh basil leaves**, and **2 tablespoons balsamic vinaigrette**. Season to taste.

EACH SERVING ABOUT: *412 calories, 18 g protein, 47 g carbohydrate, 17 g total fat (3 g saturated fat), 798 mg sodium, 458 mg calcium, 9 g fiber, 10 mg omega-3*

V

GOOD FOR: *Cancer prevention, brain, strength, hair, nails, and teeth*

GOOD FOR: *Blood sugar, brain, hair, nails, and teeth*

MAKE IT A MEAL!
Serve with
an orange.

OPEN-FACED PICKLED HERRING SANDWICH

MAKES 1 serving

In a medium bowl, whisk **1 tablespoon light sour cream** with **1 tablespoon light canola oil mayonnaise** and **1 teaspoon chopped fresh dill**. Add **½ cup pickled herring**, **¼ chopped apple**, and **1 tablespoon chopped sweet onion**. Season to taste and mix to combine. Serve on **1 slice pumpernickel bread**.

EACH SERVING ABOUT: *342 calories, 14 g protein, 29 g carbohydrate, 18 g total fat (3 g saturated fat), 960 mg sodium, 107 mg calcium, 3 g fiber, 1,030 mg omega-3*

GOOD FOR: *Heart, blood sugar, cancer prevention, brain, strength, skin, hair, nails, and teeth*

QUINOA CANNELLINI SALAD

MAKES 1 serving

Prepare **¼ cup quinoa** according to package directions. Set aside. In a medium bowl, whisk together **1 tablespoon fresh lemon juice**, **2 teaspoons extra virgin olive oil**, and **1 tablespoon chopped fresh parsley**. Toss with cooked quinoa, **½ cup rinsed and drained no-salt-added canned cannellini beans**, **½ cup chopped steamed asparagus**, and **1 tablespoon chopped walnuts**. Season to taste.

EACH SERVING ABOUT: *409 calories, 15 g protein, 50 g carbohydrate, 18 g total fat (2 g saturated fat), 57 mg sodium, 93 mg calcium, 10 g fiber, 820 mg omega-3*

SALMON PESTO SANDWICH

MAKES 1 serving

Drizzle **4 ounces grilled or drained canned salmon** with **2 teaspoons pesto**. Serve on **1 whole-wheat sandwich thin** with **2 slices of tomato** and **¼ cup baby spinach**.

EACH SERVING ABOUT: *316 calories, 35 g protein, 25 g carbohydrate, 11 g total fat (2 g saturated fat), 690 mg sodium, 190 mg calcium, 6 g fiber, 1,380 mg omega-3*

LC

GOOD FOR: *Heart, blood sugar, cancer prevention, brain, strength, skin, hair, nails, and teeth*

MAKE IT A MEAL! *Serve with* **Cantaloupe Cucumber Salad**, *recipe page 215.*

SARDINE, CUCUMBER, AND ENDIVE SANDWICH

MAKES 1 serving

In a small bowl, combine **¼ chopped, seeded cucumber**, **½ thinly sliced radish**, **¼ cup chopped endive**, **¾ teaspoon chopped fresh dill**, **¾ teaspoon white wine vinegar**, **½ teaspoon olive oil**, **¼ teaspoon sugar**, and **1½ teaspoons light sour cream**. Spread over **1 slice whole-wheat bread**. Top with **3 drained water-packed sardines** and **1 additional slice whole-wheat bread**.

EACH SERVING ABOUT: *384 calories, 27 g protein, 42 g carbohydrate, 13 g total fat (2 g saturated fat), 828 mg sodium, 170 mg calcium, 7 g fiber, 1690 mg omega-3*

GOOD FOR: *Brain, strength, hair, nails, and teeth*

MAKE IT A MEAL! *Serve with* **1 cup grape tomatoes**.

TUNA CHEDDAR MELT

MAKES 1 serving

In a small bowl, combine **2 teaspoons honey mustard**, **1 teaspoon canola oil mayonnaise**, and **3 ounces no-salt-added drained canned water-packed tuna**. Place **¼ cup baby spinach** on a **½ whole-wheat sandwich thin**. Season to taste. Top with tuna, **2 tomato slices**, and **1 thin slice cheddar cheese**. Heat under broiler for 3 minutes or until cheese melts. Top with remaining **½ sandwich thin**.

EACH SERVING ABOUT: *342 calories, 32 g protein, 26 g carbohydrate, 11 g total fat (4 g saturated fat), 434 mg sodium, 208 mg calcium, 6 g fiber, 250 mg omega-3*

TUNA FENNEL WRAP

MAKES 1 serving

In a medium bowl, whisk **1 teaspoon extra virgin olive oil** with **2 teaspoons honey mustard**. Add **3 ounces no-salt-added drained canned water-packed tuna**, **¼ apple (chopped)**, **¼ cup diced fennel**, **¼ cup chopped arugula**, **1 tablespoon dried cranberries**, and **1 tablespoon sunflower seeds**. Season to taste and mix to combine. Serve in an **8-inch whole-wheat tortilla**.

EACH SERVING ABOUT: *399 calories, 28 g protein, 39 g carbohydrate, 14 g total fat (3 g saturated fat), 459 mg sodium, 35 mg calcium, 6 g fiber, 260 mg omega-3*

VEGGIE BURGER PARMESAN

MAKES 1 serving

In a skillet sprayed with **nonstick cooking spray**, prepare **1 veggie burger** according to package directions. Serve on a **toasted whole-wheat hamburger bun** with **2 tablespoons warm marinara sauce** and **1 ounce sliced part-skim mozzarella**.

EACH SERVING ABOUT: *341 calories, 23 g protein, 35 g carbohydrate, 14 g total fat (5 g saturated fat), 994 mg sodium, 298 mg calcium, 7 g fiber, 50 mg omega-3*

LC V

GOOD FOR: *Blood sugar, cancer prevention, brain, strength, and skin*

MAKE IT A MEAL! *Serve with **1 cup arugula** drizzled with **2 teaspoons each olive oil and balsamic vinegar**. Season to taste.*

DINNER

AVOCADO CHICKEN

GF LC

GOOD FOR: *Heart, blood sugar, brain, strength, hair, nails, and teeth*

MAKES 4 main-dish servings
PREP TIME 10 minutes
COOK TIME 10 minutes

1 ripe avocado, mashed
1 tablespoon fresh lime juice
1½ tablespoons chopped fresh cilantro
4 6-ounce skinless, boneless chicken breasts
1 tablespoon olive oil
¼ teaspoon kosher salt
¼ teaspoon ground black pepper
¼ teaspoon garlic powder

1 Preheat grill or broiler to high.
2 In a medium bowl, combine avocado, lime juice, and cilantro. Set aside.
3 Brush chicken breasts with olive oil. Season with salt, pepper, and garlic powder.
4 Grill or broil 8–10 minutes or until chicken reaches an internal temperature of 165°F.
5 Remove chicken from grill. Serve topped with avocado mixture.

EACH SERVING ABOUT: *283 calories, 37 g protein, 3 g carbohydrate, 13 g total fat (2 g saturated fat), 320 mg sodium, 14 mg calcium, 2 g fiber, 90 mg omega-3*

MAKE IT A MEAL!
Serve with **1 medium baked potato** *with* **2 tablespoons nonfat plain Greek yogurt** *or* **reduced-fat sour cream***, as well as* **5 steamed asparagus spears** *drizzled with* **1 teaspoon olive oil***, per person.*

GOOD FOR: *Heart,
blood sugar, cancer
prevention, brain,
strength, skin, hair,
nails, and teeth*

BEEF STIR-FRY

MAKES 4 main-dish servings
PREP TIME 30 minutes
COOK TIME 15 minutes

MAKE IT A MEAL!
*Serve with **1 cup
asparagus** sautéed
in **1 teaspoon
canola oil**, per
person.*

1 cup brown rice

2 tablespoons cornstarch

12 ounces boneless sirloin steak, cut in thin strips

4 teaspoons canola oil, divided use

2 red bell peppers, cut into 1/2-inch strips

1 pound bok choy, stalks and leaves cut in half lengthwise,
   then cut crosswise in 1-inch pieces; separate stalks
   and leaves

4 ounces snow peas

2 tablespoons peeled fresh ginger, minced

2 cloves garlic, minced

1 teaspoon grated fresh orange peel

1/2 cup orange juice

4 teaspoons reduced-sodium soy sauce

1 tablespoon chopped pistachios

1 Cook rice according to package directions.
2 Meanwhile, place the cornstarch and beef in a resealable bag. Seal and shake to coat.
3 Heat 2 teaspoons of the oil in a large nonstick skillet over medium-high heat. Add beef and cook, stirring occasionally, until cooked through, about 3 minutes. Transfer to a plate.
4 Heat the remaining oil in the skillet and add the peppers and bok choy stalks. Cook, stirring, until almost crisp-tender, about 5 minutes. Add the bok choy leaves and snow peas and cook, stirring for 2 minutes. Push the vegetables to edge of skillet. Add the ginger and garlic in center and cook until fragrant, about 30 seconds.
5 Add orange peel and orange juice, soy sauce, and beef. Season to taste. Cook, tossing, until heated through. Top with chopped pistachios.

EACH SERVING ABOUT: *426 calories, 23 g protein, 53 g carbohydrate, 13 g total fat (3 g saturated fat), 317 mg sodium, 162 mg calcium, 5 g fiber, 530 mg omega-3*

GOOD FOR: *Heart, blood sugar, cancer prevention, brain, strength, skin, hair, nails, and teeth*

MAKE IT A MEAL!
*Serve with a salad of **½ romaine lettuce heart**, **2 large slices tomato**, and **1 tablespoon balsamic or Italian vinaigrette**, per person.*

BEET TABBOULEH WITH GRILLED CHICKEN

MAKES 4 main-dish servings
PREP TIME 30 minutes
COOK TIME 10 minutes

DRESSING
2 ½ tablespoons lemon juice
2 ½ tablespoons extra virgin olive oil
½ teaspoon Dijon mustard
½ teaspoon dried oregano
¼ teaspoon garlic, minced
Large pinch kosher salt
Ground black pepper to taste

GRILLED CHICKEN
4 6-ounce boneless, skinless chicken breasts
1 tablespoon olive oil
¼ teaspoon kosher salt
¼ teaspoon ground black pepper

TABBOULEH
¾ cup bulgur wheat
1 garlic clove, minced
2 medium raw beets, peeled and shredded
1 yellow bell pepper, finely chopped
2 scallions, thinly sliced
½ cup fresh parsley, finely chopped
⅓ cup fresh basil, finely chopped
⅓ cup fresh mint, finely chopped
¼ teaspoon kosher salt

GARNISH
Lemon wedges (optional)

1 Start tabbouleh: In a large bowl, combine bulgur, garlic, and 1 cup boiling water. Cover with large plate and let stand 30 minutes or until bulgur has softened and water is absorbed.
2 Meanwhile, preheat broiler or grill to high.
3 Make dressing: In a medium bowl, whisk together lemon juice, olive oil, Dijon mustard, dried oregano, minced garlic, salt, and pepper. Set aside.
4 Cook chicken: Brush chicken breasts with olive oil. Season with salt and pepper.
5 Grill or broil 8–10 minutes or until chicken reaches an internal temperature of 165°F. Remove from the oven or grill. Slice into ½-inch slices. Set aside.
6 Make tabbouleh: To bowl of bulgur, add beets, yellow pepper, scallions, parsley, basil, mint, dressing, and salt. Stir until well combined.
7 Assemble: Top tabbouleh with sliced chicken. Serve with lemon wedges, if desired.

EACH SERVING ABOUT: *437 calories, 41 g protein, 30 g carbohydrate, 17 g total fat (3 g saturated fat), 558 mg sodium, 72 mg calcium, 8 g fiber, 150 mg omega-3*

GOOD FOR: *Heart, blood sugar, cancer prevention, brain, strength, skin, hair, nails, and teeth*

ADD ON DESSERT! *Spray **2 ½-inch pineapple slices** per person with **nonstick cooking spray** and grill on each side for 3 minutes.*

CASHEW-CHICKEN STIR-FRY

MAKES 4 main-dish servings
PREP TIME 10 minutes
COOK TIME 10 minutes

1 cup instant brown rice
1 cup reduced-sodium chicken broth
2 tablespoons reduced-sodium soy sauce
1 tablespoon brown sugar
1 tablespoon cornstarch
2 teaspoons canola oil
1 pound chicken tenders, cut crosswise if large
12 ounces broccoli florets
1 medium red pepper, cut into 1-inch pieces
1 small onion, cut in half and sliced
1 teaspoon peeled fresh ginger, minced
½ cup cashews
1 teaspoon Asian sesame oil

1 Prepare rice according to package directions. Set aside.
2 In a small bowl, stir together broth, soy sauce, sugar, and cornstarch.
3 Meanwhile, in a nonstick skillet, heat canola oil over medium-high heat until hot. Add chicken and cook 4–5 minutes or until it just loses its pink color throughout, stirring frequently. Transfer chicken to bowl.
4 To same skillet, add broccoli, red pepper, onion, ginger, and ¼ cup broth mixture. Cover skillet and cook 3 minutes or until vegetables are tender-crisp, stirring occasionally. Stir remaining broth mixture. Add broth mixture and chicken with any juices to skillet. Heat to boiling. Boil 1 minute or until mixture thickens slightly.
5 Remove skillet from heat. Stir in cashews and sesame oil. Season to taste.
6 Top rice with chicken mixture.

EACH SERVING ABOUT: *411 calories, 33 g protein, 37 g carbohydrate, 16 g total fat (3 g saturated fat), 377 mg sodium, 60 mg calcium, 5 g fiber, 390 mg omega-3*

GOOD FOR: *Cancer prevention, strength, skin, hair, nails, and teeth*

CAULIFLOWER CURRY STEW

MAKES 4 main-dish servings
PREP TIME 10 minutes
COOK TIME 20 minutes

3 medium red potatoes, cut into ½-inch chunks
⅓ cup plus 2 tablespoons water, divided use
1 head cauliflower, cut into ½-inch chunks
1½ tablespoons canola oil, divided use
1 sweet onion, finely chopped
3 cloves garlic, minced
1 tablespoon peeled, minced fresh ginger
1½ teaspoons ground cumin
2 15-ounce cans no-salt-added chickpeas, rinsed and drained
1 14.5-ounce can fire-roasted tomatoes
½ teaspoon ground turmeric
Large pinch cayenne pepper (or more, to taste, up to
      ¼ teaspoon)
½ teaspoon kosher salt
¼ cup chopped fresh cilantro leaves
1 cup nonfat plain Greek yogurt

1 In a large microwave-safe bowl, combine potatoes and
   2 tablespoons water. Cover with vented plastic wrap and
   microwave on high 5 minutes.

2 Uncover bowl. Add cauliflower, cover with vented plastic wrap,
   and microwave on high 5 minutes or until just tender. Remove
   from microwave and drain.

3 Meanwhile, in a large skillet, heat 1 tablespoon canola oil
   over medium-high heat until hot. Add onion; cook 2–3 minutes
   or until golden brown and tender, stirring occasionally. Add
   garlic, ginger, and cumin. Cook 30 seconds or until golden,
   stirring.

4 Add remaining ½ tablespoon canola oil, then potatoes and
   cauliflower. Cook 3 minutes and lightly brown, stirring to coat.
   Stir in chickpeas, tomatoes, turmeric, cayenne, and remaining
   ⅓ cup water.

5 Heat to boiling, and then reduce heat to medium and simmer
   4 minutes or until tender, stirring and scraping up any brown
   bits. Stir in salt. Remove from heat. Top with cilantro and
   yogurt.

EACH SERVING ABOUT: *496 calories, 24 g protein, 85 g carbohydrate,
7 g total fat (0 g saturated fat), 621 mg sodium, 209 mg calcium, 16 g fiber,
500 mg omega-3*

CAULIFLOWER MAC 'N' CHEESE

V

GOOD FOR: *Cancer prevention, brain, strength, skin, hair, nails, and teeth*

MAKES 4 main-dish servings
PREP TIME 10 minutes
COOK TIME 50 minutes

MAKE IT A MEAL!
Serve with
***1 medium tomato**, sliced and drizzled with **1 teaspoon** **balsamic vinegar**, per person.*

1 head cauliflower, cut into 1-inch florets, stems discarded
4 medium carrots, thinly sliced
1 cup reduced-sodium vegetable broth
¼ cup reduced-fat cream cheese
1 teaspoon Dijon mustard
1 pinch cayenne pepper
¾ cup shredded Gruyère cheese
¼ teaspoon kosher salt
¼ teaspoon ground black pepper
10 ounces elbow macaroni
3 cups small broccoli florets
2 plum tomatoes, cored, seeded, and chopped
¼ cup grated Parmesan cheese

1 Preheat oven to 400°F.

2 Heat an 8-quart saucepot of water to boiling on high. Add cauliflower and carrots to boiling water. Cook 15 minutes or until very tender.

3 Meanwhile, in a blender, combine broth, cream cheese, mustard, cayenne, Gruyère, salt, and pepper.

4 With slotted spoon, transfer vegetables to blender, reserving water. Blend vegetables until puréed.

5 Add pasta to reserved boiling water. Cook for half the time that the label directs, adding broccoli during last minute of cooking.

6 Drain pasta and broccoli and return to pot. Stir in cauliflower sauce and half of tomatoes.

7 Spread in 2½-quart shallow baking dish. Top with tomatoes and Parmesan.

8 Bake 35 minutes or until golden brown on top and heated through.

EACH SERVING ABOUT: *479 calories, 24 g protein, 72 g carbohydrate, 12 g total fat (6 g saturated fat), 507 mg sodium, 383 mg calcium, 9 g fiber, 190 mg omega-3*

CHICKEN VEGETABLE SKEWERS

MAKES 4 main-dish servings
PREP TIME 25 minutes
COOK TIME 15 minutes

2 tablespoons fresh lemon juice
2 tablespoons olive oil
2 garlic cloves, minced
2 teaspoons chopped fresh rosemary
¼ teaspoon kosher salt
¼ teaspoon ground black pepper
1 pound skinless, boneless chicken breast, cut into 1-inch cubes
2 cups grape tomatoes
2 zucchini, cut into ½-inch slices
24 brown or cremini mushrooms, trimmed
1 cup instant brown rice

1 In a large bowl, whisk together lemon juice, olive oil, garlic, rosemary, salt, and pepper. Add chicken, tomatoes, zucchini, and mushrooms. Mix well to combine. Cover and refrigerate for 15 minutes.

2 Meanwhile, prepare rice according to package directions. Set aside.

3 Preheat grill or broiler to high.

4 Remove chicken and vegetables from refrigerator. Thread on 12 large skewers.

5 Grill for 8–10 minutes, turning halfway through cooking time.

6 Serve over rice.

EACH SERVING ABOUT: *336 calories, 31 g protein, 29 g carbohydrate, 11 g total fat (2 g saturated fat), 276 mg sodium, 55 mg calcium, 4 g fiber, 90 mg omega-3*

CURRIED RICE WITH SHRIMP AND PEAS

MAKES 4 main-dish servings
PREP TIME 5 minutes
COOK TIME 30 minutes

GOOD FOR: *Cancer prevention, brain, strength, skin, hair, nails, and teeth*

1 tablespoon olive oil
1 large onion, finely chopped
¼ teaspoon kosher salt
⅛ teaspoon ground black pepper
1½ tablespoons peeled fresh ginger, minced
2 cloves garlic, minced
1 tablespoon curry powder
1 cup long-grain white rice
2 cups water
1 pound medium shrimp, peeled and deveined
1 cup frozen peas, thawed
1 cup fresh cilantro, chopped
Lemon wedges for serving (optional)

MAKE IT A MEAL!
*Serve with **1 serving of Cumin-Spiced Pumpkin Soup** per person (recipe on page 217).*

1 In a large skillet, heat the oil over medium heat. Add the onion, season with salt and pepper. Cook, covered, stirring occasionally, until tender, 6–8 minutes.
2 Add the ginger and garlic and cook, stirring, for 2 minutes. Add the curry powder and cook, stirring, for 1 minute.
3 Add the rice and stir to coat. Stir in 2 cups water and bring to a boil. Reduce the heat and simmer, covered, for 15 minutes.
4 Fold the shrimp and peas into the partially cooked rice and cook, covered, until the shrimp is opaque throughout and the rice is tender, 4–5 minutes more.
5 Remove from heat and fold in the cilantro.
6 Serve with lemon wedges, if desired.

EACH SERVING ABOUT: *331 calories, 21 g protein, 48 g carbohydrate, 5 g total fat (1 g saturated fat), 769 mg sodium, 96 mg calcium, 3 g fiber, 100 mg omega-3*

CORKSCREW PASTA WITH SAUSAGE AND FENNEL

MAKES 4 main-dish servings
PREP TIME 10 minutes
COOK TIME 45 minutes

1 small fennel bulb
5 ounces hot Italian sausage links
10 ounces corkscrew or rotelle macaroni
¼ teaspoon kosher salt
4 teaspoons olive oil
1½ medium carrots, cut into ¼-inch round slices
½ medium onion, diced
1 28-ounce can Italian plum tomatoes
1 tablespoon chopped parsley (optional)

1 Rinse fennel with cold water. Cut off and discard root end and stalks. Cut bulb in half through root end. Then place each half cut-side down and thinly slice lengthwise. Remove casings from sausages.

2 In a large stockpot, prepare corkscrew macaroni in boiling water according to package directions. Drain, reserving ½ cup pasta cooking water. Return pasta to saucepot; keep warm.

3 Meanwhile, in a large skillet over medium-high heat, cook sausage until browned, stirring frequently to break up sausage. Remove sausage to medium bowl. To drippings in skillet, add fennel and salt, stirring frequently, until fennel is tender-crisp and begins to brown. Remove to bowl with sausage; keep warm.

4 In same skillet, warm olive oil over medium heat. Add carrots and onion and cook until tender. Add tomatoes with their liquid and reserved pasta cooking water, stirring to break up tomatoes. Bring to a boil. Reduce heat to low and simmer, uncovered, 10 minutes.

5 Stir tomato sauce into pasta in saucepot. Spoon pasta onto platter. Top with sausage and fennel. Sprinkle with chopped parsley, if desired. Toss before serving.

EACH SERVING ABOUT: *490 calories, 17 g protein, 68 g carbohydrate, 17 g total fat (5 g saturated fat), 845 mg sodium, 85 mg calcium, 6 g fiber, 150 mg omega-3*

FARMERS MARKET PASTA

MAKES 4 main-dish servings
PREP TIME 15 minutes
COOK TIME 15 minutes

8 ounces whole-wheat linguine
¼ cup olive oil
2 cloves garlic, minced
1 large pinch crushed red pepper flakes
¼ cup white wine (or reduced-sodium chicken or vegetable broth)
1 tablespoon Dijon mustard
1 teaspoon lemon zest
2 tablespoons lemon juice
¼ teaspoon kosher salt
¼ teaspoon ground black pepper
2 cups frozen lima beans, cooked in microwave
2 zucchini, cut into thin ribbons
½ pound asparagus, cut into 1-inch pieces and steamed
¼ cup grated Parmesan cheese

1 In a large pot of boiling water, prepare linguine according to package directions. Drain pasta.
2 Meanwhile, in a large sauté pan, heat olive oil over medium-low heat. Add garlic and red pepper and sauté 1 minute. Add white wine and cook for 1 minute more.
3 Remove sauté pan from heat. Whisk in mustard, lemon zest, lemon juice, salt, and pepper.
4 Add lima beans, zucchini, asparagus, and cooked pasta. Toss well. Top with grated Parmesan to serve.

EACH SERVING ABOUT: *498 calories, 19 g protein, 70 g carbohydrate, 17 g total fat (3 g saturated fat), 541 mg sodium, 153 mg calcium, 14 g fiber, 90 mg omega-3*

GREEK-STYLE TILAPIA

MAKES 4 main-dish servings
PREP TIME 10 minutes
COOK TIME 20 minutes

1 cup whole-wheat couscous
2 lemons
Nonstick cooking spray
4 6-ounce tilapia fillets
1 tablespoon fresh oregano leaves, chopped
¼ teaspoon kosher salt
¼ teaspoon ground black pepper
1 pint grape tomatoes, halved

1 Preheat oven to 400°F.
2 Prepare couscous according to package directions. Set aside.
3 Meanwhile, from lemons, grate ½ teaspoon peel and squeeze ¼ cup juice.
4 Spray a 9x13-inch glass or ceramic baking dish with nonstick cooking spray. Arrange tilapia fillets in baking dish. Evenly sprinkle fillets with lemon juice and peel, oregano, salt, and pepper. Add tomatoes to baking dish around tilapia. Cover with foil and roast 16–18 minutes or until tilapia is opaque throughout and tomatoes are tender.
5 Serve tilapia, tomatoes, and couscous with juices from baking dish.

EACH SERVING ABOUT: *354 calories, 42 g protein, 41 g carbohydrate, 4 g total fat (1 g saturated fat), 212 mg sodium, 51 mg calcium, 7 g fiber, 290 mg omega-3*

GOOD FOR: *Heart, blood sugar, cancer prevention, brain, strength, skin, hair, nails, and teeth*

GLUTEN-FREE VERSION: *Swap in **1 cup quinoa or brown rice** for whole-wheat couscous.*

MAKE IT A MEAL! *Serve with **¾ cup microwaved frozen peas** tossed with **1 teaspoon olive oil**, per person.*

ADD ON DESSERT! ***1 serving of Watermelon Granita** per person (recipe on page 221).*

GARLIC SHRIMP AND SWISS CHARD ON POLENTA

MAKES 4 main-dish servings
PREP TIME 20 minutes
COOK TIME 20 minutes

2 cups water
1 cup 1% milk
¼ teaspoon kosher salt
3 tablespoons extra virgin olive oil, divided use
1 pound large shrimp, peeled and deveined
1 medium red onion, halved and cut into thin strips
2 cloves garlic, minced
**1 pound Swiss chard, stems cut into 2-inch strips,
    leaves torn into large pieces and all rinsed**
1 14.5-ounce can no-salt-added tomatoes, undrained
¼ teaspoon ground black pepper
1 cup instant polenta
1 tablespoon unsalted butter
¼ cup grated Parmesan cheese

1 In a medium saucepan, combine water, milk, and salt. Slowly bring to a boil over medium-low heat.

2 Meanwhile, in a large, deep nonstick skillet, heat 2 tablespoons of the oil to medium-high heat. Add shrimp and red onion. Sauté 2 minutes. Add garlic and continue to sauté 1 minute, just until shrimp turns opaque and onion is almost translucent. Remove mixture to a plate.

3 Add remaining 1 tablespoon oil to skillet and sauté chard stems over medium heat for 2 minutes. Top with chard leaves; cover skillet with lid, and cook 1 minute until leaves are wilted. Uncover and continue to sauté 2 minutes. Add tomatoes with their juice and simmer 4 minutes. Season with pepper.

4 Bring water-milk mixture to a full boil. Slowly whisk in polenta until smooth. Cook over medium-low heat 3 minutes, stirring until thick and creamy. Remove from heat. Stir in butter and cheese.

5 Raise heat on chard mixture and add shrimp mixture. Cook 2 to 3 minutes longer, until shrimp are cooked through. Serve shrimp mixture on polenta.

EACH SERVING ABOUT: *469 calories, 27 g protein, 53 g carbohydrate, 17 g total fat (5 g saturated fat), 1,131 mg sodium, 279 mg calcium, 7 g fiber, 180 mg omega-3*

GOOD FOR: *Heart, blood sugar, cancer prevention, brain, strength, skin, hair, nails, and teeth*

MAKE IT A MEAL!
Serve with **1/2 cup warmed rinsed and drained no-salt-added canned black beans** *per person.*

GRILLED CHICKEN SALAD WITH AVOCADO AND GRAPEFRUIT

MAKES 4 main-dish servings
PREP TIME 10 minutes
COOK TIME 10 minutes

DRESSING

3 tablespoons fresh grapefruit juice, reserved when sectioning grapefruit for salad (below)
1½ tablespoons fresh lemon juice
1½ tablespoons chopped fresh cilantro
1½ teaspoons honey
¼ teaspoon kosher salt
¼ teaspoon ground black pepper
1 tablespoon olive oil

GRILLED CHICKEN

4 6-ounce boneless, skinless chicken breasts
¼ teaspoon kosher salt
¼ teaspoon ground black pepper
¼ teaspoon chili powder

SALAD

4 large romaine lettuce leaves
2 avocados, peeled, pitted and thinly sliced
2 pink grapefruits, peeled, sectioned over a bowl to catch juices for dressing
¼ medium red onion, thinly sliced

1 Make the dressing: In a small bowl, whisk together grapefruit and lemon juices, cilantro, honey, salt, and pepper. Slowly whisk in olive oil. Set aside.
2 Cook the chicken: Preheat grill or broiler to high.
3 Season chicken with salt, pepper, and chili powder.
4 Grill or broil 8–10 minutes or until chicken reaches an internal temperature of 165°F. Set aside.
5 Divide dressing in half. Toss half with the grilled chicken. Reserve remaining dressing for salad.
6 Make the salad: Line four salad plates with lettuce. Fan avocado and grapefruit on lettuce and top with onion. Drizzle with remaining dressing. Place chicken on the side.

EACH SERVING ABOUT: *422 calories, 39 g protein, 27 g carbohydrate, 18 g total fat (3 g saturated fat), 444 mg sodium, 68 mg calcium, 8 g fiber, 130 mg omega-3*

LEMON PASTA WITH SALMON AND ASPARAGUS

MAKES 4 main-dish servings
PREP TIME 15 minutes
COOK TIME 25 minutes

2 5-ounce salmon fillets
1/2 teaspoon kosher salt, divided use
1/4 teaspoon ground black pepper, divided use
8 ounces whole-wheat penne pasta
3 cups fresh asparagus, cut into 1-inch pieces
1/4 cup olive oil
2 cloves garlic, thinly sliced
2 tablespoons shallots, finely minced
1/4 cup fresh lemon juice
1/4 cup reduced-sodium chicken broth
1/4 cup fresh basil, chopped

1 Preheat broiler. Season salmon with 1/4 teaspoon salt and 1/8 teaspoon pepper. Place salmon on broiling pan and broil for 8–10 minutes, or until just cooked through. Remove from oven. Cut salmon into 1-inch chunks. Set aside.

2 Bring a large stockpot of water to a boil. Add pasta and prepare according to package directions. Three minutes before pasta is cooked, add asparagus and continue to cook. Drain and set aside.

3 In a large sauté pan, heat olive oil over medium-low heat. Add garlic and shallot. Sauté for 2 minutes. Add lemon juice, chicken broth, and remaining 1/4 teaspoon salt and 1/8 teaspoon pepper. Bring to a boil. Reduce heat to low and simmer 2 more minutes. Remove from heat. Add cooked pasta and asparagus and salmon chunks. Toss well. Sprinkle pasta with basil.

EACH SERVING ABOUT: *472 calories, 25 g protein, 49 g carbohydrate, 21 g total fat (3 g saturated fat), 300 mg sodium, 60 mg calcium, 7 g fiber, 870 mg omega-3*

LEMON SHRIMP

MAKES 4 main-dish servings
PREP TIME 15 minutes
COOK TIME 15 minutes

¼ cup lemon juice
4 teaspoons Dijon mustard
4 teaspoons minced garlic
¼ teaspoon kosher salt
⅛ teaspoon freshly ground black pepper
1 pound large shrimp, peeled and deveined
8 ounces angel hair pasta
¼ cup olive oil
¼ cup fresh parsley, chopped

1 In a medium bowl, whisk lemon juice, mustard, garlic, salt, and pepper together. Add shrimp and marinate for 10 minutes.
2 While shrimp marinates, prepare pasta in a large pot of boiling water according to package directions. Drain.
3 In a large sauté pan, heat olive oil over medium heat. Add shrimp and marinade and cook, stirring frequently until shrimp turns opaque, about 5 minutes.
4 Pour shrimp and juices over pasta and toss. Top with parsley.

EACH SERVING ABOUT: *418 calories, 23 g protein, 46 g carbohydrate, 17 g total fat (2 g saturated fat), 888 mg sodium, 85 mg calcium, 2 g fiber, 80 mg omega-3*

GOOD FOR: *Brain, strength, hair, nails, and teeth*

MAKE IT A MEAL! *Serve with **1 cup cooked string beans** drizzled with **1 teaspoon olive oil** and **1 teaspoon balsamic vinegar**, per person.*

LINGUINE WITH CHICKEN, SPINACH, AND MUSHROOMS

MAKES 4 main-dish servings
PREP TIME 20 minutes
COOK TIME 25 minutes

10 ounces linguine
1 tablespoon olive oil
8 ounces boneless, skinless chicken breast,
   cut into thin strips
1/2 teaspoon kosher salt, divided use
1 medium onion, diced
8 ounces shiitake or brown mushrooms, thinly sliced
1 1/4 cups reduced-sodium chicken broth
6 ounces reduced-fat cream cheese
1 medium bunch spinach, cleaned, stems removed and
   coarsely chopped
1/4 teaspoon ground black pepper

1 In a large stockpot, bring water to a boil. Prepare linguine according to package directions. Drain.

2 Meanwhile, in a large skillet, heat olive oil over medium-high heat. Add chicken. Season with 1/4 teaspoon salt. Cook until lightly browned and chicken just loses its color, about 5 minutes. Transfer chicken to a bowl.

3 Add onion to skillet and cook until almost tender, about 5 minutes. Add mushrooms and remaining salt. Cook until mushrooms and onions are golden, about 5 minutes.

4 Add chicken broth and cream cheese. Raise heat to high and heat until boiling, stirring until cream cheese melts. Boil for 2 minutes. Stir in chicken, spinach, and pepper, and heat through. Toss linguine with chicken mixture.

EACH SERVING ABOUT: *480 calories, 30 g protein, 64 g carbohydrate, 12 g total fat (5 g saturated fat), 602 mg sodium, 250 mg calcium, 5 g fiber, 130 mg omega-3*

LINGUINE WITH TOMATOES, SPINACH, AND CLAMS

GOOD FOR: *Heart, cancer prevention, strength, skin, hair, nails, and teeth*

MAKES 4 main-dish servings
PREP TIME 10 minutes
COOK TIME 15 minutes

8 ounces linguine
¼ cup olive oil
6 cloves garlic, minced
½ teaspoon crushed red pepper flakes
1 14.5-ounce can crushed tomatoes
¾ cup white wine (or reduced-sodium vegetable broth)
2 6.5-ounce cans chopped clams, drained
¼ cup chopped parsley
1 bunch spinach, stems discarded
¼ cup grated Parmesan cheese

1 In a large stockpot, prepare pasta according to package directions. Drain.
2 Meanwhile, in a large skillet, heat the oil, garlic, and crushed red pepper over medium heat, stirring occasionally, 2–3 minutes.
3 Add tomatoes, wine, and clams to skillet, stirring occasionally for 5 minutes. Stir in the parsley. Add the pasta and spinach and toss. Season to taste. Top with grated Parmesan.

EACH SERVING ABOUT: *480 calories, 21 g protein, 57 g carbohydrate, 17 g total fat (3 g saturated fat), 1,007 mg sodium, 201 mg calcium, 6 g fiber, 130 mg omega-3*

GOOD FOR: *Heart,
blood sugar, cancer
prevention, brain,
strength, skin, hair,
nails, and teeth*

MEDITERRANEAN SHRIMP AND BULGUR

MAKES 4 main-dish servings
PREP TIME 35 minutes
COOK TIME 10 minutes

1 cup bulgur
1 cucumber, diced
4 scallions, sliced
½ cup fresh mint, chopped
12 ounces frozen cooked large shrimp, thawed
2 cups grape tomatoes, halved
⅓ cup lemon juice
¼ cup extra virgin olive oil
4 cups arugula, roughly chopped
¼ cup crumbled feta cheese

1 Place bulgur in a medium bowl. Add 2 cups boiling water to
   cover and soak 30 minutes. Drain well.
2 Return bulgur to bowl. Add cucumber, scallion, mint, shrimp,
   tomatoes, lemon juice, olive oil, and arugula. Season to taste.
   Toss well. Sprinkle with feta.

EACH SERVING ABOUT: *364 calories, 20 g protein, 36 g carbohydrate,
17 g total fat (3 g saturated fat), 555 mg sodium, 158 mg calcium, 9 g fiber,
120 mg omega-3*

PASTA WITH ASPARAGUS, CANNELLINI, AND PARMESAN

V

GOOD FOR: *Heart, blood sugar, cancer prevention, brain, strength, skin, hair, nails, and teeth*

MAKES 4 main-dish servings
PREP TIME 10 minutes
COOK TIME 15 minutes

8 ounces whole-wheat penne pasta
¼ cup olive oil
4 cups chopped asparagus
4 cloves garlic, thinly sliced
2 cups rinsed and drained no-salt-added canned cannellini beans
2 cups chopped tomatoes
½ cup reduced-sodium vegetable broth
¼ teaspoon kosher salt
¼ teaspoon ground black pepper
¼ cup chopped fresh basil
3 tablespoons grated Parmesan cheese

1 In a large pot of boiling water, prepare pasta according to package directions. Drain.
2 Meanwhile, in a large skillet, heat olive oil over medium-low heat. Add asparagus and sauté for 3 minutes. Add garlic and sauté for 1 additional minute.
3 Reduce heat to low. Add cooked pasta, cannellini beans, tomatoes, vegetable broth, salt, and pepper. Toss well. Remove from heat.
4 Top with basil and Parmesan.

EACH SERVING ABOUT: *500 calories, 19 g protein, 70 g carbohydrate, 18 g total fat (3 g saturated fat), 253 mg sodium, 155 mg calcium, 14 g fiber, 30 mg omega-3*

GOOD FOR: *Brain,
strength, skin, hair,
nails, and teeth*

MEDITERRANEAN STEAK SALAD

MAKES 4 main-dish servings
PREP TIME 15 minutes
COOK TIME 15 minutes

1 teaspoon dried oregano
1 teaspoon garlic powder
¼ teaspoon cinnamon
¼ teaspoon kosher salt
¼ teaspoon ground black pepper
¼ cup extra virgin olive oil
¼ cup balsamic vinegar
12 ounces flank steak, visible fat trimmed
Nonstick cooking spray
1 red bell pepper, cored
8 cups mixed salad greens
1 large tomato, cut into eighths
¼ cup sliced black olives, drained
4 large whole-wheat pita breads, warmed

1 Preheat grill or broiler to high.
2 In a small bowl, make a spice rub by mixing oregano, garlic powder, cinnamon, salt, and pepper together.
3 Reserving remaining rub for later, whisk 1 teaspoon rub in a small bowl with olive oil and balsamic vinegar. Set aside.
4 Divide remaining rub in half. Sprinkle steak with half of reserved spice rub to season on all sides. Spray red pepper with cooking spray. Sprinkle red pepper with remaining half of spice rub.
5 Grill or broil pepper for 7 minutes. Add steak to grill or broiler, and cook 4–6 minutes on each side. Remove steak and pepper to a cutting board. Let steak rest for 5 minutes. Cut pepper into ½-inch strips.
6 Meanwhile, place salad greens, tomato, olives, and red peppers into a large bowl. Thinly slice steak across the grain and add to salad. Drizzle with dressing and toss well. Serve with warmed whole-wheat pitas.

EACH SERVING ABOUT: *492 calories, 27 g protein, 48 g carbohydrate, 23 g total fat (4 g saturated fat), 561 mg sodium, 48 mg calcium, 9 g fiber, 180 mg omega-3*

MEXICAN BURRITO BOWL

MAKES 4 main-dish servings
PREP TIME 10 minutes
COOK TIME 10 minutes

2 cups instant brown rice
1 tablespoon olive oil
1 red bell pepper, thinly sliced
1 yellow bell pepper, thinly sliced
1 large yellow onion, thinly sliced
2 cloves garlic, thinly sliced
1 cup frozen corn, thawed
¼ teaspoon dried thyme
¼ teaspoon kosher salt
¼ teaspoon ground black pepper
3 cups rinsed and drained no-salt-added canned pinto beans
2 cups shredded lettuce
2 large tomatoes, diced
1 avocado, diced
½ cup salsa
Lime wedges for serving (optional)

1 In a medium stockpot, prepare rice according to package directions. Set aside.
2 Meanwhile, in a large saucepan, heat olive oil to medium-low heat. Add red and yellow peppers and onions and sauté 5 minutes. Add garlic and sauté 2 minutes more. Add corn, thyme, salt, and pepper, and sauté 2 additional minutes. Remove from heat.
3 In a microwave-safe container, microwave pinto beans until just heated through, about 2 minutes. Stir well.
4 Divide rice among four serving bowls. Top each equally with heated vegetables, pinto beans, lettuce, tomatoes, and avocado.
5 Serve with salsa and lime wedges, if desired.

EACH SERVING ABOUT: *508 calories, 17 g protein, 87 g carbohydrate, 11 g total fat (1 g saturated fat), 396 mg sodium, 133 mg calcium, 18 g fiber, 90 mg omega-3*

ORANGE-SOY TOFU STIR-FRY

MAKES 4 main-dish servings
PREP TIME 10 minutes
COOK TIME 15 minutes

3/4 cup water
1 teaspoon orange zest
1/4 cup orange juice
2 tablespoons reduced-sodium soy sauce
1 1/2 teaspoons cornstarch
1/4 teaspoon crushed red pepper flakes
2 teaspoons canola oil, divided use
1 14-ounce package extra-firm tofu, patted dry, cut into 1-inch cubes
2 teaspoons garlic, minced
2 teaspoons peeled fresh ginger, minced
1 pound asparagus, cut into 1-inch pieces
2 medium red peppers, sliced
1 cup frozen shelled edamame
3 1/2 ounces sliced shiitake mushrooms
1/2 cup sliced scallions
4 tablespoons sesame seeds

1 Mix water, orange zest, orange juice, soy sauce, cornstarch, and crushed red pepper flakes in a small bowl.

2 In a large nonstick skillet, heat 1 teaspoon oil over high heat. Add tofu and cook until golden, turning often, about 5 minutes. Add garlic and ginger. Reduce heat and cook 30 seconds. Remove from skillet.

3 Add remaining 1 teaspoon oil to skillet. Add asparagus, peppers, edamame, and mushrooms. Fry, stirring frequently 5 minutes.

4 Add orange juice mixture and bring to boil. Stir in tofu and scallions. Season to taste. Toss and top with sesame seeds.

EACH SERVING ABOUT: *278 calories, 19 g protein, 22 g carbohydrate, 14 g total fat (0 g saturated fat), 320 mg sodium, 303 mg calcium, 8 g fiber, 240 mg omega-3*

GOOD FOR: *Heart,*
blood sugar, cancer
prevention, brain,
strength, skin, hair,
nails, and teeth

GLUTEN-FREE
VERSION: *Omit*
soy sauce and
substitute **a gluten-**
free tamari sauce.

MAKE IT A MEAL!
Serve with
¼ cup brown rice
prepared according
to package
directions per
person.

PEPPER-CRUSTED TUNA
WITH SESAME ASPARAGUS

MAKES 4 main-dish servings
PREP TIME 10 minutes
COOK TIME 10 minutes

1 pound asparagus, cut into 1-inch pieces
2 tablespoons sesame oil
2 tablespoons reduced-sodium soy sauce
2 tablespoons sesame seeds
4 5-ounce tuna steaks
1 teaspoon freshly ground black pepper
Nonstick cooking spray

1 In a medium pot of boiling water, cook asparagus for
   5 minutes. Drain. Toss with sesame oil, soy sauce, and
   sesame seeds. Set aside.
2 Meanwhile, sprinkle tuna steaks with black pepper to
   season on all sides.
3 Spray a skillet or grill pan with nonstick cooking spray
   and heat over medium-high heat. Add tuna and cook for
   4–6 minutes, flipping halfway through the cooking time.
   Remove from pan. Serve with asparagus.

EACH SERVING ABOUT: *324 calories, 37 g protein, 6 g carbohydrate,*
17 g total fat (3 g saturated fat), 354 mg sodium, 55 mg calcium, 3 g fiber,
1,910 mg omega-3

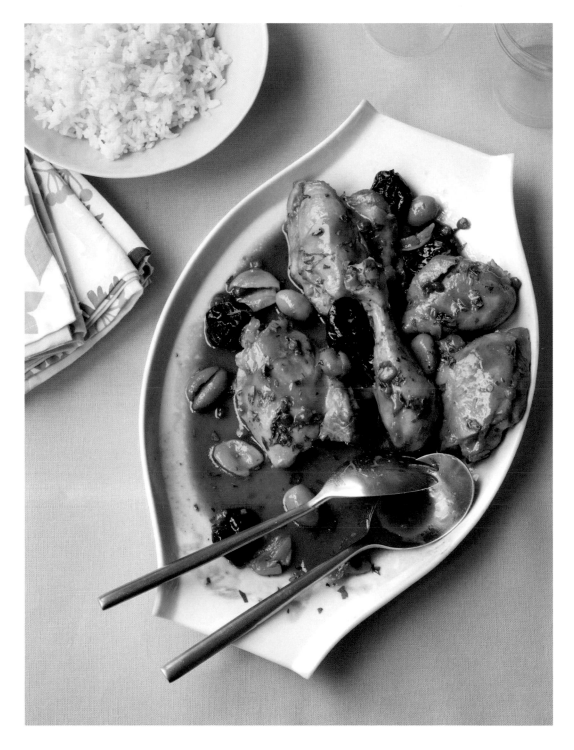

Slow Cooker Chicken Marbella (recipe on page 198)

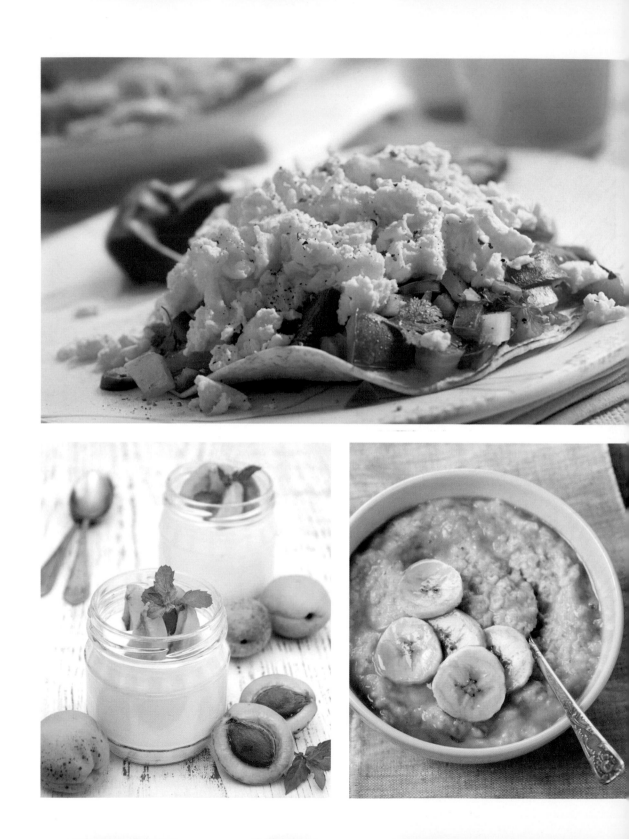

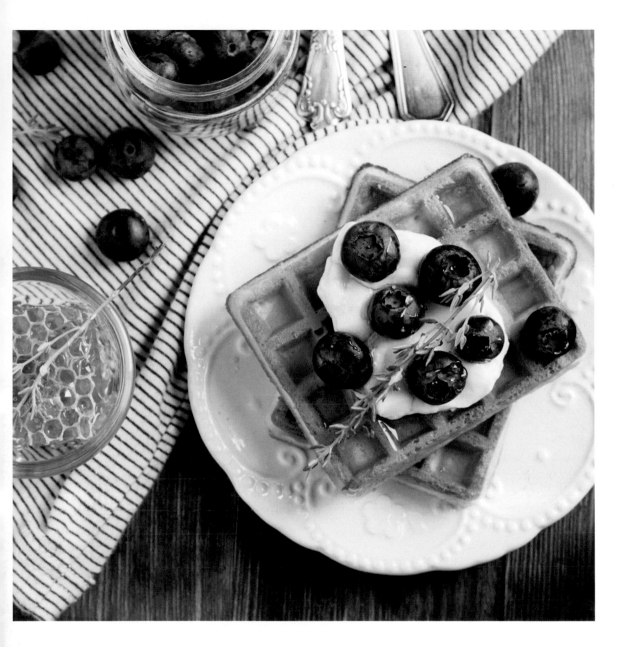

CLOCKWISE, FROM UPPER LEFT: *Huevos Rancheros (recipe on page 140), PB & Banana Oatmeal (recipe on page 142), Apricot Ricotta Breakfast Sundae (recipe on page 137)*
ABOVE: *Better-For-You Blueberry Waffles (recipe on page 137)*

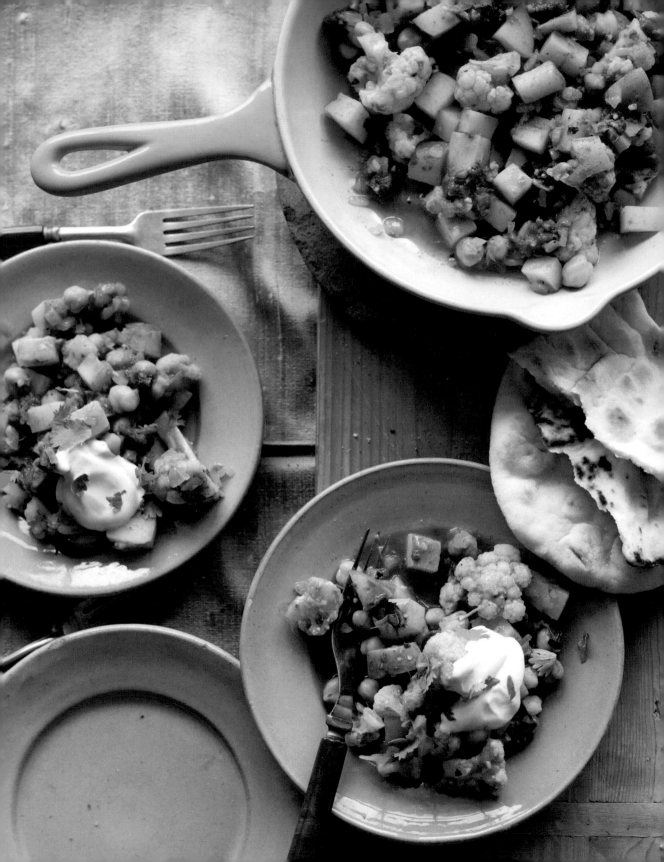

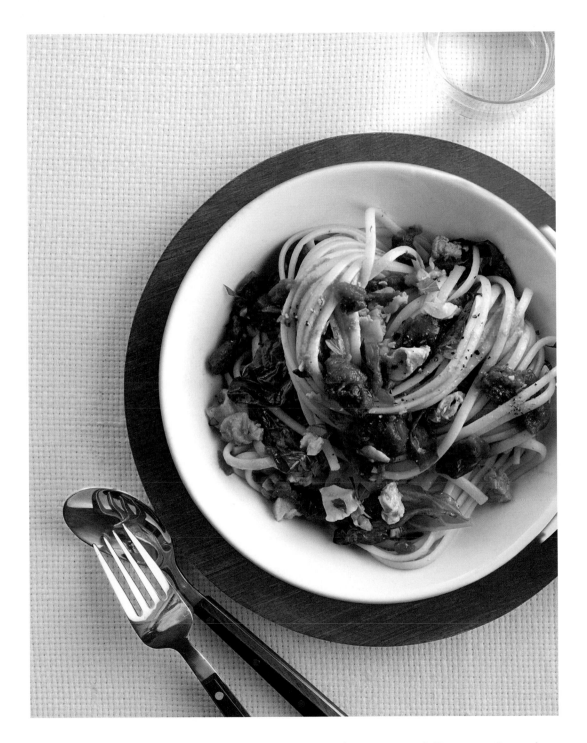

FROM LEFT: *Cauliflower Curry Stew (recipe on page 166), Linguine with Tomatoes, Spinach, and Clams (recipe on page 183)*

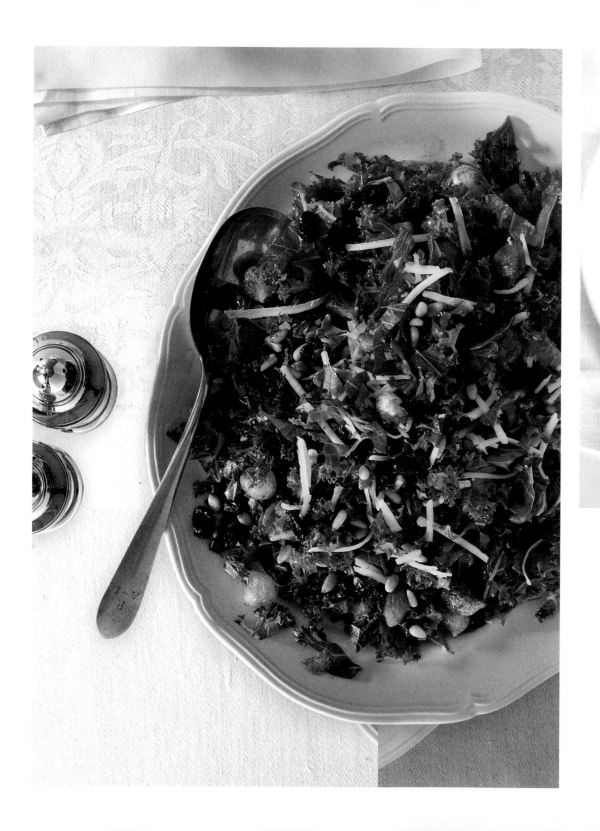

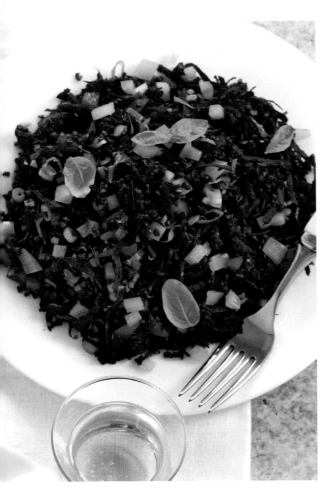

FROM LEFT: *Kale Salad with Chicken and Cheddar (recipe on page 153), Beet Tabbouleh with Grilled Chicken (recipe on page 162), Steak and Onion Tacos with Fresh Tomato Salsa (recipe on page 206)*

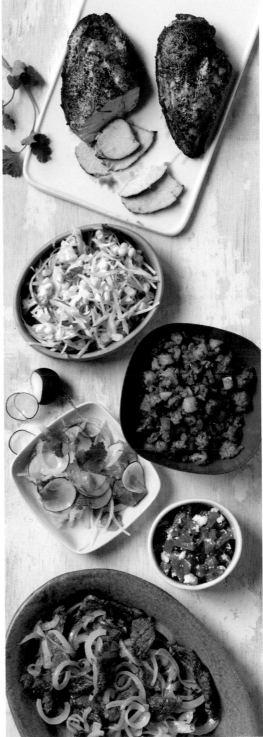

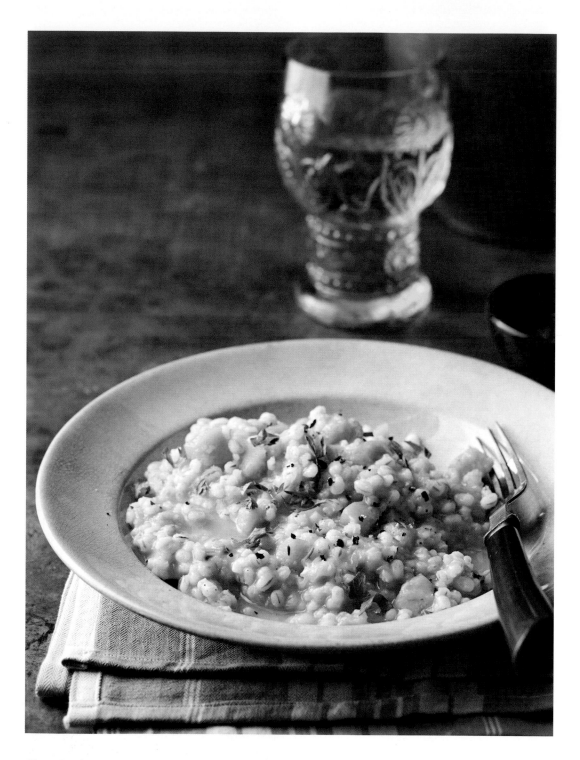

Slow Cooker Butternut Squash Barley Risotto (recipe on page 197)

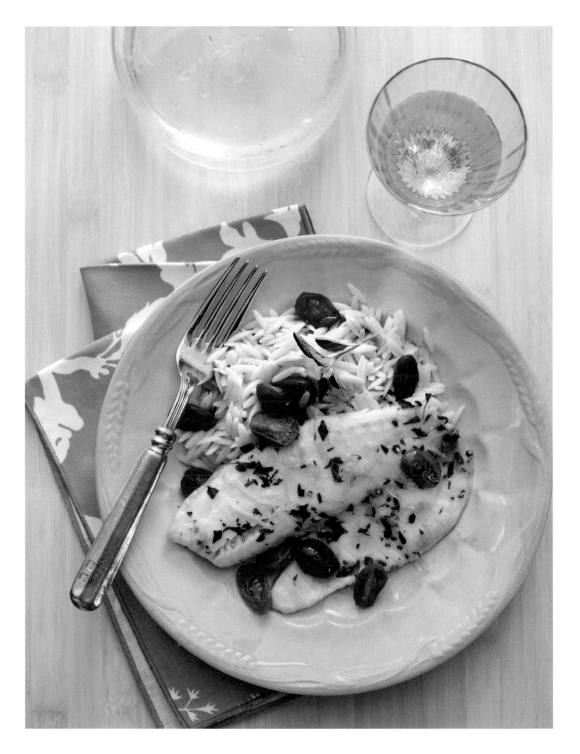

Greek-Style Tilapia (recipe on page 175)

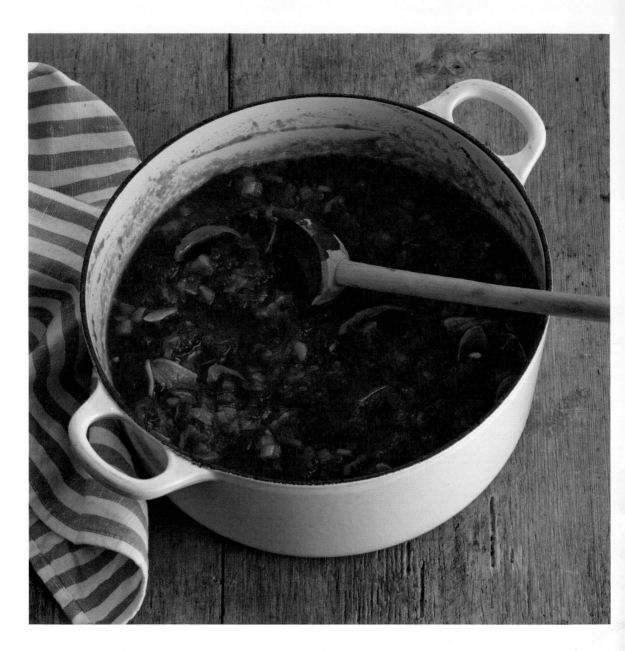

ABOVE: *Summer Tomato Sauce (recipe on page 220)*
RIGHT, CLOCKWISE, FROM TOP: *Cauliflower Mac 'n' Cheese (recipe on page 168), Quinoa Cannellini Salad (recipe on page 154), Cantaloupe Cucumber Salad (recipe on page 215)*

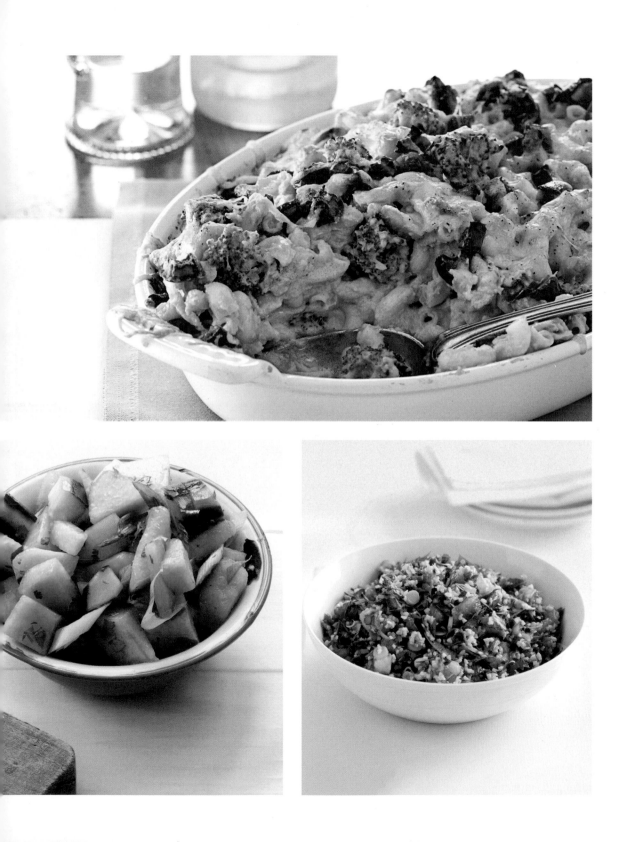

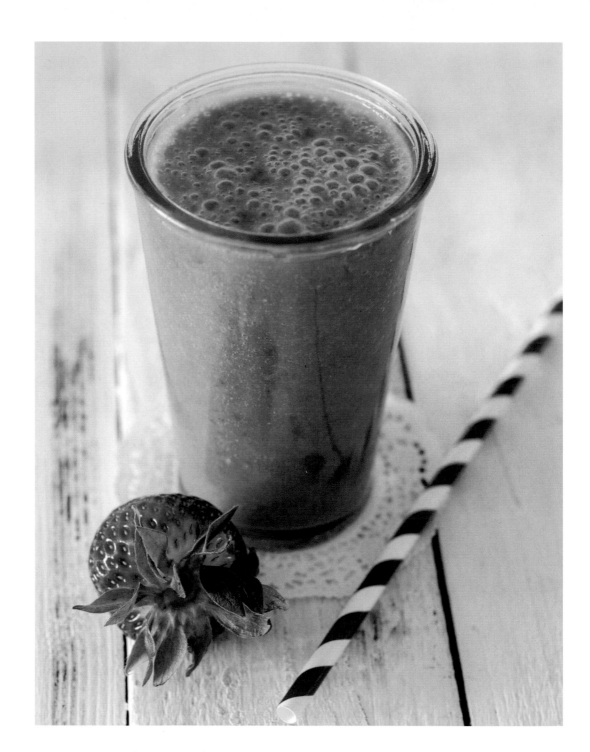

FROM LEFT: *Strawberry Smoothie (recipe on page 226), Walnut-Crusted Chicken Cutlets (recipe on page 209)*

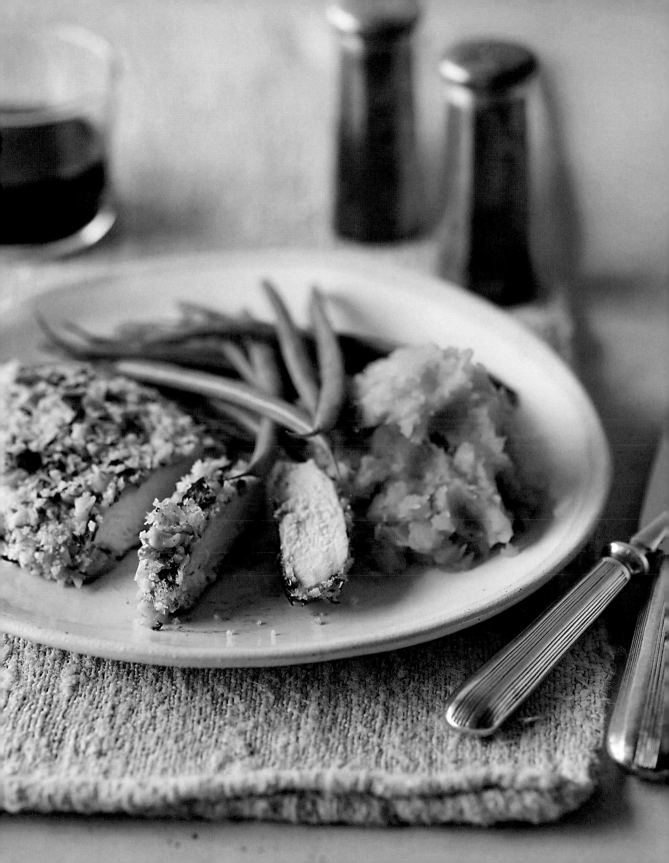

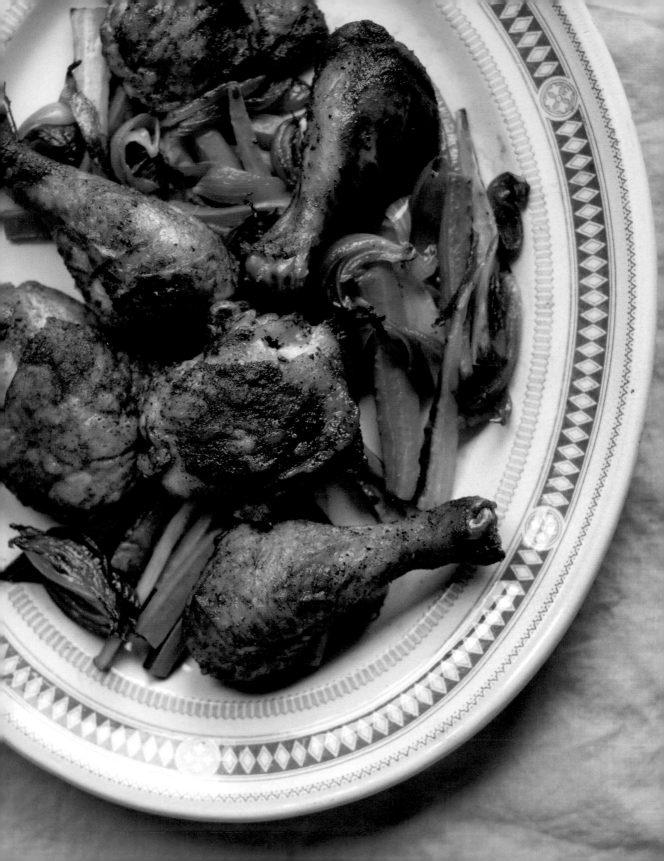

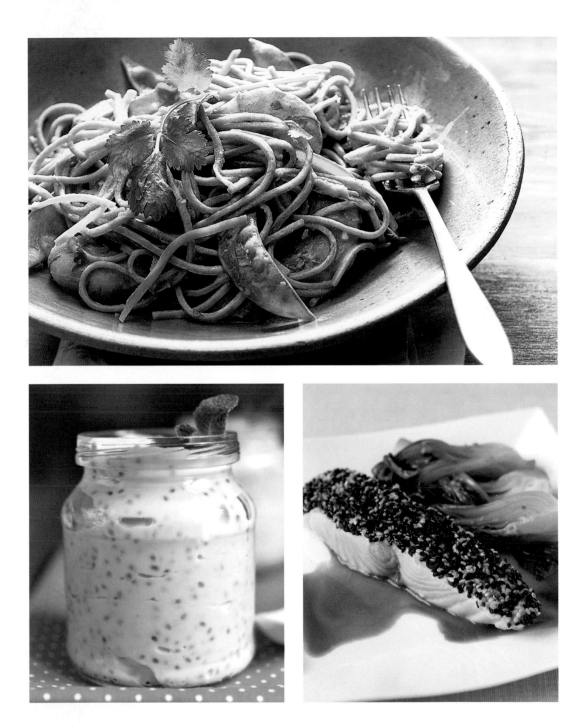

LEFT: *Spice Roasted Chicken, Red Onions, Carrots, and Parsnips (recipe on page 204)*
ABOVE, CLOCKWISE, FROM TOP: *Soba Noodles with Shrimp, Snow Peas, Carrots, and Edamame (recipe on page 200), Sesame Salmon with Bok Choy (recipe on page 195), Chia Pudding (recipe on page 224)*

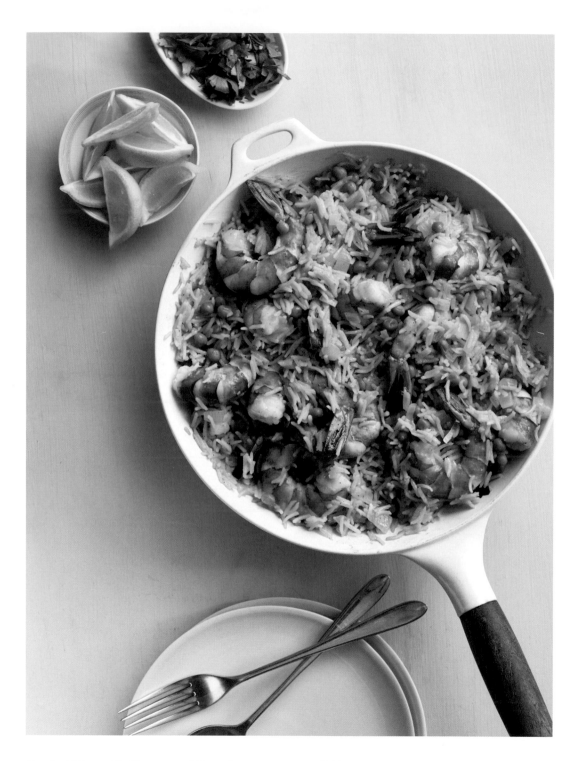

Curried Rice with Shrimp and Peas (recipe on page 171)

ROAST PORK TENDERLOIN WITH BLACKBERRY SAUCE

MAKES 4 main-dish servings
PREP TIME 15 minutes
COOK TIME 35 minutes

1¼ pounds pork tenderloin
1 teaspoon garlic powder
1 teaspoon dried rosemary
2 teaspoons canola oil
2²/3 cups fresh blackberries
2 tablespoons plus 2 teaspoons Worcestershire sauce
2 tablespoons balsamic vinegar
2 tablespoons tomato paste
¼ cup water
½ teaspoon ground mustard
Large pinch cayenne pepper

1 Preheat oven to 450°F.
2 Season pork with garlic powder and rosemary.
3 In a large skillet, heat canola oil over medium-high heat. Add pork and sear for 10 minutes, turning frequently.
4 Remove pork from skillet and transfer to a roasting pan. Roast for 20 minutes or until pork reaches an internal temperature of 145°F. Remove from oven.
5 Meanwhile, in a medium saucepan, combine blackberries, Worcestershire, balsamic vinegar, tomato paste, water, mustard, and cayenne pepper. Bring to a simmer over medium heat. Simmer 5–7 minutes or until berries have softened, stirring occasionally.
6 Slice pork and top with berry sauce.

EACH SERVING ABOUT: *249 calories, 31 g protein, 13 g carbohydrate, 8 g total fat (2 g saturated fat), 224 mg sodium, 43mg calcium, 6 g fiber, 330 mg omega-3*

LC

GOOD FOR: *Heart, blood sugar, cancer prevention, brain, strength, skin, hair, nails, and teeth*

GLUTEN-FREE VERSION: *Omit Worcestershire sauce or choose* **a gluten-free Worcestershire sauce**.

MAKE IT A MEAL! *Serve with* **¼ cup whole-wheat couscous** *prepared according to package directions, and* **½ cup broccoli florets** *sautéed in* **1 teaspoon olive oil**, *per person. To make this gluten-free, substitute* **¼ cup quinoa or brown rice** *for couscous.*

SALMON CAKES

MAKES 4 main-dish servings
PREP TIME 10 minutes
COOK TIME 10 minutes

MAKE IT A MEAL!
*Serve on **a whole-wheat hamburger bun** with **lettuce**, **tomato**, and **1 tablespoon cocktail sauce**, per person, plus a salad of **1 cup arugula**, **¼ cup rinsed and drained no-salt-added canned cannellini beans**, and **1 tablespoon balsamic vinaigrette**, per person.*

1 14 ¾-ounce can red or pink salmon, drained and flaked
1 egg, lightly beaten
1 scallion, sliced
3 tablespoons prepared horseradish
2 tablespoons plain dried breadcrumbs
1 teaspoon reduced-sodium soy sauce
¼ teaspoon ground black pepper
Nonstick cooking spray

1 In a medium bowl, lightly mix all ingredients except cooking spray with a fork. Shape mixture into 4 3-inch round patties. Spray both sides of patties with cooking spray.
2 Heat a large skillet over medium heat. Add salmon cakes, and cook about 5 minutes per side or until golden.

EACH SERVING ABOUT: *185 calories, 28 g protein, 4 g carbohydrate, 6 g total fat (1 g saturated fat), 535 mg sodium, 82 mg calcium, 1 g fiber, 1,240 mg omega-3*

SESAME SALMON WITH BOK CHOY

MAKES 4 main-dish servings
PREP TIME 10 minutes
COOK TIME 25 minutes

4 5-ounce salmon fillets
¼ teaspoon ground black pepper
3 tablespoons sesame seeds
¼ cup reduced-sodium soy sauce
1 garlic clove, minced
1 teaspoon minced fresh ginger
½ teaspoon sesame oil
Large pinch crushed red pepper flakes
2 bunches (about 1½ pounds) bok choy,
    cut crosswise into thirds and root ends quartered
1 teaspoon unsalted butter

1 Preheat oven to 375°F.
2 On waxed paper, sprinkle salmon with pepper to season all sides. Coat 1 side of each salmon fillet with sesame seeds.
3 Heat a large oven-safe skillet over medium-high heat. Add salmon, sesame seed side down, and cook 2 minutes (do not turn). Transfer skillet to oven and bake salmon 10–12 minutes or just until salmon turns opaque in center.
4 Meanwhile, in a medium saucepan, combine soy sauce, garlic, ginger, sesame oil, and crushed red pepper.
5 Add bok choy to soy sauce mixture. Toss to combine. Cover and heat to boiling over high heat. Reduce heat to medium and cook, covered, 8 minutes, stirring occasionally. Uncover and cook 3 minutes longer or until bok choy is tender.
6 Remove saucepot from heat. Discard garlic. Gently stir butter into soy-sauce mixture until blended. Serve salmon, seed side up, with bok choy and drizzle with soy-sauce mixture.

EACH SERVING ABOUT: *320 calories, 37 g protein, 12 g carbohydrate, 15 g total fat (2 g saturated fat), 923 mg sodium, 482 mg calcium, 5 g fiber, 3,210 mg omega-3*

LC

GOOD FOR: *Blood sugar, cancer prevention, brain, strength, skin, hair, nails, and teeth*

GLUTEN-FREE VERSION: *Omit soy sauce and substitute **a gluten-free tamari sauce**.*

MAKE IT A MEAL! *Serve with **¼ cup brown rice** prepared according to package directions per person.*

GF V

GOOD FOR: *Heart, cancer prevention, brain, strength, skin, hair, nails, and teeth*

SLOW COOKER AFRICAN SWEET POTATO–PEANUT STEW

MAKES 4 main-dish servings
PREP TIME 25 minutes
COOK TIME 8 hours

2 cloves garlic
1 1/3 cup fresh cilantro leaves and stems
1 15.5-ounce can diced tomatoes, undrained
1/3 cup creamy or chunky peanut butter
1 1/2 teaspoons ground cumin
1/2 teaspoon ground cinnamon
Large pinch cayenne pepper
1/4 teaspoon kosher salt
2/3 cup water
2 pounds sweet potatoes, peeled and cut into 2-inch chunks
1 15.5-ounce can no-salt-added chickpeas, rinsed and drained
10 ounces frozen green beans, thawed

1 In blender or food processor with knife blade attached, blend garlic, cilantro, tomatoes with their juice, peanut butter, cumin, cinnamon, cayenne pepper, and salt until puréed.
2 Pour mixture into 4 1/2- to 6-quart slow cooker bowl. Stir in water. Add sweet potatoes and chickpeas. Stir to combine. Cover slow cooker with lid and cook on low setting 8 to 10 hours or on high setting 4 to 5 hours or until potatoes are very tender.
3 About 10 minutes before sweet potato mixture is done, cook green beans as label directs. Gently stir green beans into stew.

EACH SERVING ABOUT: *490 calories, 17 g protein, 81 g carbohydrate, 12 g total fat (2 g saturated fat), 598 mg sodium, 176 mg calcium, 16 g fiber, 50 mg omega-3*

SLOW COOKER BUTTERNUT SQUASH BARLEY RISOTTO

v

GOOD FOR: *Heart, cancer prevention, brain, and skin*

MAKES 4 main-dish servings
PREP TIME 15 minutes
COOK TIME 3 hours 45 minutes

1 tablespoon olive oil
1 shallot, thinly sliced
1 sprig fresh thyme
1 cup pearl barley
2 cups reduced-sodium vegetable broth
1 cup water
1 pound butternut squash, cut into 1/2-inch cubes
1/2 teaspoon kosher salt, divided use
1/4 teaspoon ground black pepper
1/4 cup grated Parmesan cheese
1 tablespoon chopped fresh parsley

1   In a 12-inch skillet, heat olive oil over medium-high heat. Add shallot and cook 2 minutes or until golden, stirring often. Add thyme; cook 30 seconds. Add barley and cook 2 minutes or until toasted and golden, stirring often.

2   Transfer to a 4 1/2- to 6-quart slow cooker, along with broth, water, squash, and 1/4 teaspoon salt. Cover and cook on high for 3 1/2–4 hours or until liquid is absorbed and squash is tender.

3   Uncover and discard thyme. Add Parmesan, remaining 1/4 teaspoon salt, and pepper. Gently stir until Parmesan melts. Garnish with parsley.

EACH SERVING ABOUT: *318 calories, 9 g protein, 58 g carbohydrate, 6 g total fat (1 g saturated fat), 393 mg sodium, 115 mg calcium, 10 g fiber, 10 mg omega-3*

SLOW COOKER CHICKEN MARBELLA

GOOD FOR: *Blood sugar, brain, strength, skin, hair, nails, and teeth*

MAKE IT A MEAL! *Serve with **1 cup cooked string beans** drizzled with **1 teaspoon olive oil** and **1 teaspoon balsamic vinegar**, per person.*

MAKES 4 main-dish servings
PREP TIME 15 minutes
COOK TIME 3–6 hours

½ cup dry white wine (or reduced-sodium chicken or vegetable broth)
2 tablespoons brown sugar
1½ teaspoons dried oregano
3 tablespoons red wine vinegar, divided use
¼ teaspoon kosher salt
¼ teaspoon ground black pepper
6 cloves garlic, smashed
1 tablespoon capers
½ cup dried plums
8 green olives
4 skinless chicken legs, split into 4 drumsticks and 4 thighs
¼ cup chopped parsley

1 In a 5–6–quart slow cooker bowl, whisk together wine, brown sugar, oregano, 2 tablespoons of vinegar, salt, and pepper. Add garlic, capers, dried plums, and olives. Mix to combine.
2 Add chicken, nesting it among olives and dried plums. Cover and cook on low until meat is tender and cooked through, 5–6 hours or high for 3–4 hours. Gently stir in remaining 1 tablespoon vinegar and parsley.

EACH SERVING ABOUT: *446 calories, 52 g protein, 23 g carbohydrate, 13 g total fat (3 g saturated fat), 620 mg sodium, 50 mg calcium, 1 g fiber, 180 mg omega-3*

SLOW COOKER ITALIAN LENTIL AND VEGETABLE STEW

MAKES 4 main-dish servings
PREP TIME 10 minutes
COOK TIME 8–10 hours

1¼ cups dried lentils, rinsed
2½ cups diced butternut squash
1⅔ cups marinara sauce
2 cups green beans, cut in half
¾ medium red bell pepper, cut in 1-inch pieces
1 medium potato, peeled and cut in 1-inch pieces
1 clove garlic, minced
⅔ cup chopped onion
2½ teaspoons extra virgin olive oil
¼ cup grated Parmesan cheese

1 Mix lentils and 2½ cups of water in a 3-quart (or larger) slow cooker.
2 In a large bowl, mix remaining ingredients except olive oil and Parmesan.
3 Cover and cook on low 8–10 hours until the vegetables are tender.
4 Stir in olive oil and top with Parmesan.

EACH SERVING ABOUT: *426 calories, 20 g protein, 74 g carbohydrate, 8 g total fat (2 g saturated fat), 567 mg sodium, 188 mg calcium, 17 g fiber, 190 mg omega-3*

V

GOOD FOR: *Heart, cancer prevention, brain, strength, skin, hair, nails, and teeth*

ADD ON DESSERT!
½ cup sliced strawberries mixed with ½ cup pomegranate seeds, per person.

SOBA NOODLES WITH SHRIMP, SNOW PEAS, CARROTS, AND EDAMAME

MAKES 4 main-dish servings
PREP TIME 15 minutes
COOK TIME 10 minutes

¼ cup creamy peanut butter
2 teaspoons peeled minced fresh ginger
2 tablespoons reduced-sodium soy sauce
1 tablespoon distilled white vinegar
1 teaspoon sesame oil
½ teaspoon hot sauce
8 ounces soba noodles
1½ cups shredded carrots
1½ cups frozen shelled edamame, thawed
1 pound large shrimp, shelled and deveined
4 ounces snow peas, strings removed
½ cup fresh cilantro, chopped, plus extra for garnish

1 In a small bowl, place peanut butter, ginger, soy sauce, vinegar, sesame oil, and hot sauce. Set aside.
2 Bring a medium stockpot of water to a boil over high heat. Add noodles and cook 4 minutes. Add carrots and edamame and cook 1 minute. Add shrimp and snow peas and cook 2 minutes more.
3 Reserve ½ cup pasta cooking water. Drain noodles, shrimp, and vegetables into large colander. Transfer noodle mixture to large bowl.
4 Whisk reserved cooking water into peanut butter mixture until well blended. Add peanut sauce and chopped cilantro leaves to noodle mixture in bowl and toss until evenly coated. Garnish with cilantro.

EACH SERVING ABOUT: *488 calories, 35 g protein, 56 g carbohydrate, 14 g total fat (2 g saturated fat), 1,351 mg sodium, 147 mg calcium, 8 g fiber, 80 mg omega-3*

SPAGHETTI WITH BEETS, GREENS, AND RICOTTA

GOOD FOR: *Cancer prevention, brain, strength, skin, hair, nails, and teeth*

MAKES 4 main-dish servings
PREP TIME 25 minutes
COOK TIME 25 minutes

2 bunches beets with tops (about 3 pounds)
8 ounces whole-wheat spaghetti
3 tablespoons olive oil
2 cloves garlic, minced
Large pinch crushed red pepper
½ teaspoon kosher salt
1 cup part-skim ricotta cheese

1 Cut tops from beets and reserve. If beets are not uniform in size, cut larger beets in half. Place beets and ½ cup water in deep 3-quart microwave-safe baking dish. Cover and cook in microwave oven on high 15–20 minutes or until beets are tender when pierced with the tip of a knife. Rinse beets under cold running water until cool enough to handle. Peel beets and cut into ½-inch pieces.

2 Meanwhile, in large saucepot of boiling water, prepare spaghetti according to package directions, reserving ¾ cup of the pasta cooking water. Drain.

3 Trim stems from beet tops. Coarsely chop beet greens and set greens aside.

4 In a large nonstick skillet, heat oil, garlic, and crushed red pepper over medium heat for 2 minutes or until garlic is lightly golden. Increase heat to medium-high. Add beet greens to skillet, and cook 3 minutes, stirring. Add cooked beets and salt. Cook 1–2 minutes or until mixture is heated through.

5 Return spaghetti to saucepot. Add beet mixture, ricotta, and reserved pasta cooking water and toss well.

EACH SERVING ABOUT: *498 calories, 22 g protein, 73 g carbohydrate, 17 g total fat (5 g saturated fat), 755 mg sodium, 363 mg calcium, 17 g fiber, 80 mg omega-3*

MAKE IT A MEAL!
*Serve with **¼ cup quinoa** prepared according to package directions and **1 cup broccoli** sautéed in **2 teaspoons olive oil**, per person.*

SPICED PORK TENDERLOINS WITH MANGO SALSA

MAKES 4 main-dish servings
PREP TIME 20 minutes
COOK TIME 5 minutes

SALSA
1 ripe mango, peeled and coarsely chopped
1 kiwi, peeled and coarsely chopped
1 tablespoon rice vinegar
1½ teaspoons peeled minced fresh ginger
1½ teaspoons chopped fresh cilantro leaves

PORK
1 pound whole pork tenderloin
1½ tablespoons all-purpose flour
¼ teaspoon kosher salt
½ teaspoon ground cumin
½ teaspoon ground coriander
¼ teaspoon ground cinnamon
¼ teaspoon ground ginger

1 Prepare salsa: In a medium bowl, combine mango, kiwi, vinegar, ginger, and cilantro. Set aside.

2 Prepare pork: Pre-heat grill to medium.

3 Meanwhile, cut pork tenderloin lengthwise almost in half, being careful not to cut all the way through. Open and spread flat. Place tenderloin between two sheets of plastic wrap. With a meat mallet or rolling pin, pound to ¼-inch thickness. Cut tenderloin into 4 pieces.

4 On waxed paper, mix flour, salt, cumin, coriander, cinnamon, and ground ginger. Add pork to spice mixture and turn to coat evenly.

5 Place pork on hot grill rack. Cover grill and cook pork 5–6 minutes or until lightly browned on both sides and pork just loses its pink color throughout, turning pork over once. Remove from heat. Serve with salsa.

EACH SERVING ABOUT: *211 calories, 25 g protein, 18 g carbohydrate, 5 g total fat (1 g saturated fat), 181 mg sodium, 26 mg calcium, 2 g fiber, 60 mg omega-3*

GOOD FOR: *Heart, blood sugar, cancer prevention, brain, strength, skin, hair, nails, and teeth*

ADD ON DESSERT!
1 serving of Watermelon Granita per person (recipe on page 221).

SPICE-ROASTED CHICKEN, RED ONIONS, CARROTS, AND PARSNIPS

MAKES 4 main-dish servings
PREP TIME 15 minutes
COOK TIME 35 minutes

2 medium red onions, cut into ½-inch wedges
1½ pounds medium carrots, cut into 3-inch sticks
½ pound medium parsnips, cut into 3-inch sticks
2 tablespoons olive oil
¼ teaspoon kosher salt, divided use
¼ teaspoon ground black pepper, divided use
4 chicken drumsticks
2 teaspoons paprika
1 teaspoon ground cinnamon

1 Preheat oven to 425°F.
2 On a large rimmed baking sheet, toss the onions, carrots, parsnips, olive oil, and half of the salt and pepper.
3 Season the chicken with the paprika, cinnamon, and remaining salt and pepper. Nestle the chicken pieces among the vegetables and roast for 30 to 35 minutes, until the chicken is cooked through and the vegetables are golden brown and tender.

EACH SERVING ABOUT: *411 calories, 26 g protein, 33 g carbohydrate, 20 g total fat (4 g saturated fat), 384 mg sodium, 112 mg calcium, 9 g fiber, 160 mg omega-3*

SPICY ASIAN LETTUCE WRAPS

(LC)

MAKES 4 main-dish servings
PREP TIME 10 minutes
COOK TIME 10 minutes

1 tablespoon canola oil
12 ounces 93% lean ground turkey
2 tablespoons reduced-sodium soy sauce
2 tablespoons rice wine vinegar
4 teaspoons hoisin sauce
1 8-ounce can sliced water chestnuts, drained
¼ teaspoon red pepper flakes
4 scallions, sliced
12 iceberg lettuce leaves
¼ cup chopped peanuts

1 In a large pan, heat canola oil over medium heat. Add turkey and sauté for 5 minutes
2 Add soy sauce, rice wine vinegar, hoisin sauce, water chestnuts, and red pepper flakes. Sauté 5 minutes. Remove from heat.
3 Add scallions and mix well. Season to taste. Divide among lettuce leaves. Top with chopped peanuts.

EACH SERVING ABOUT: *237 calories, 21 g protein, 10 g carbohydrate, 14 g total fat (3 g saturated fat), 379 mg sodium, 26 mg calcium, 3 g fiber, 360 mg omega-3*

GOOD FOR: *Heart, blood sugar, cancer prevention, strength, skin, hair, nails, and teeth*

MAKE IT A MEAL! *Serve with **¼ cup brown rice** cooked according to package directions.*

ADD ON DESSERT! *Enjoy **½ ounce dark chocolate** per person.*

MAKE IT A MEAL!
Serve with
3/4 cup warmed rinsed and drained no-salt-added canned black beans *per person.*

STEAK AND ONION TACOS WITH FRESH TOMATO SALSA

MAKES 4 main-dish servings
PREP TIME 15 minutes
COOK TIME 15 minutes

SALSA
4 plum tomatoes, seeded and cut into 1/4-inch pieces
1 small jalapeño, seeded and finely chopped
2 tablespoons fresh lime juice
1/4 teaspoon kosher salt
Large pinch ground black pepper
2 tablespoons chopped fresh cilantro
2 tablespoons crumbled feta cheese

TACOS
1 tablespoon olive oil
1 large yellow onion, sliced
1 teaspoon ground cumin
1/2 teaspoon chipotle chili powder
1/4 teaspoon kosher salt
1 pound sirloin steak, cut into 1-inch long strips
8 6-inch corn tortillas, warmed

1 Make salsa: In a medium bowl, toss the tomatoes, jalapeño, lime juice, salt, and pinch pepper. Fold in cilantro and cheese. Set aside.

2 Make tacos: Heat the oil in a large skillet over medium heat. Add the onion and cook, covered, stirring occasionally, until tender, 6–8 minutes.

3 Meanwhile, in a medium bowl, combine the cumin, chili powder, and salt. Add the steak and toss to coat.

4 Add the steak to the skillet with the onions, increase the heat to medium-high, and cook, tossing occasionally, until the steak is just cooked through, 3–4 minutes.

5 Spoon steak onto warmed tortillas. Serve with salsa.

EACH SERVING ABOUT: *344 calories, 24 g protein, 30 g carbohydrate, 14 g total fat (4 g saturated fat), 343 mg sodium, 33 mg calcium, 5 g fiber, 10 mg omega-3*

TURKEY CUTLETS PICCATA

MAKES 4 main-dish servings

PREP TIME 5 minutes

COOK TIME 15 minutes

½ cup all purpose flour
¼ teaspoon kosher salt
Large pinch ground black pepper
4 4-ounce turkey cutlets
¼ cup olive oil
½ cup reduced-sodium chicken broth
⅓ cup lemon juice
1 tablespoon lemon zest
3 tablespoons capers

1 In a pie plate or shallow baking dish, combine flour, salt, and pepper. Dredge turkey cutlets in flour and place on a large plate.

2 In a large skillet, heat olive oil over medium-high heat. Add turkey cutlets. Cook for 6 minutes, flipping halfway through the cooking time. Remove turkey from pan.

3 Reduce heat to low. Add chicken broth, lemon juice, and lemon zest. Cook for 5 minutes. Add capers and mix well. Return turkey to pan. Cook for 1 additional minute and serve.

EACH SERVING ABOUT: *277 calories, 29 g protein, 8 g carbohydrate, 15 g total fat (2 g saturated fat), 408 mg sodium, 7 mg calcium, 1 g fiber, 20 mg omega-3*

WALNUT-CRUSTED CHICKEN CUTLETS

LC

MAKES 4 main-dish servings
PREP TIME 15 minutes
COOK TIME 10 minutes

Nonstick cooking spray
1/3 cup panko bread crumbs
Large pinch cayenne pepper
1/4 teaspoon kosher salt
1/4 teaspoon ground black pepper
1/3 cup walnuts, toasted and cooled
2 tablespoons chopped fresh parsley
1 egg white
3/4 teaspoon Dijon mustard
1 pound chicken breast cutlets, thinly sliced

1   Preheat oven to 450°F. Place a rack in a rimmed baking sheet. Spray rack with cooking spray.
2   On a large dinner plate, combine panko, cayenne, salt, and pepper.
3   In a food processor with knife blade attached, blend walnuts and parsley until nuts are finely chopped. Toss with panko mixture until well blended. Set aside.
4   In a pie plate, whisk egg white and mustard until well blended.
5   Dip each chicken cutlet into egg white mixture and then into walnut mixture to coat 1 side. Arrange chicken on rack in baking sheet, coated side up. Spray lightly with cooking spray.
6   Bake chicken 10–12 minutes or until topping is golden brown.

EACH SERVING ABOUT: *226 calories, 27 g protein, 7 g carbohydrate, 10 mg total fat (1 g saturated fat), 300 mg sodium, 19 mg calcium, 1 g fiber, 910 mg omega-3*

GOOD FOR: *Heart, blood sugar, brain, strength, skin, hair, nails, and teeth*

MAKE IT A MEAL!
*Serve with **Carrots with Grapes and Dill** (recipe on page 216) and **1/4 cup quinoa** prepared according to package directions, per person.*

ZITI WITH EGGPLANT AND RICOTTA

V

GOOD FOR: *Heart, cancer prevention, brain, strength, skin, hair, nails, and teeth*

MAKES 4 main-dish servings
PREP TIME 10 minutes
COOK TIME 50 minutes

1 pound eggplant, cut into 1-inch pieces
2 tablespoons olive oil, divided use
1/2 teaspoon kosher salt, divided use
1 small onion, finely chopped
1 1/2 garlic cloves, minced
1 15.5-ounce can plum tomatoes in juice
4 teaspoons tomato paste
Large pinch ground black pepper
2 tablespoons fresh basil leaves, chopped, divided use
10 ounces ziti or penne pasta
3 tablespoons grated Parmesan cheese
2/3 cup part-skim ricotta cheese

1 Preheat oven to 450°F.

2 In large bowl, toss eggplant, 1½ tablespoons of the olive oil, and ¼ teaspoon of the salt until evenly coated. Arrange eggplant in a single layer on two large rimmed baking sheets. Place baking sheets with eggplant on two oven racks in oven. Roast eggplant 30 minutes or until eggplant is tender and golden, rotating pans between upper and lower racks halfway through cooking and stirring twice. Remove pans with eggplant from oven. Set aside. Lower oven temperature to 400°F.

3 Meanwhile, in medium saucepan, heat remaining ½ tablespoon olive oil to medium heat. Add onion and cook until tender, about 5 minutes, stirring occasionally. Add garlic and cook 1 minute longer, stirring frequently.

4 Stir in tomatoes with their juice, tomato paste, pepper, and remaining ¼ teaspoon salt, breaking up tomatoes with side of spoon. Heat to boiling over high heat. Reduce heat to low and simmer, uncovered, 10 minutes or until sauce thickens slightly. Stir in 1 tablespoon basil.

5 In a large saucepot, prepare pasta in boiling water according to package directions. Drain. Return pasta to saucepot.

6 To pasta in saucepot, add roasted eggplant, tomato sauce, and Parmesan. Toss until evenly mixed. Spoon mixture into a shallow casserole. Top with dollops of ricotta.

7 Cover casserole with foil and bake 20 minutes or until hot and bubbly. To serve, sprinkle with remaining 1 tablespoon basil.

EACH SERVING ABOUT: *461 calories, 18 g protein, 70 g carbohydrate, 13 g total fat (4 g saturated fat), 546 mg sodium, 222 mg calcium, 8 g fiber, 60 mg omega-3*

MAKE IT A MEAL!
Serve with **1 medium baked sweet potato** *per person.*

ZESTY APRICOT ROAST PORK MEDALLIONS

MAKES 4 main-dish servings
PREP TIME 5 minutes
COOK TIME 6 minutes

1¼ pounds pork tenderloin, cut into 1-inch medallions
¼ teaspoon kosher salt
¼ teaspoon ground black pepper
¼ cup olive oil
¼ cup apricot jam
½ cup orange juice
4 teaspoons Dijon mustard

1 Season pork with salt and pepper.
2 In a large skillet, heat olive oil over medium-high heat. Add pork medallions. Cook for 2 minutes per side. Remove from pan.
3 Remove pan from heat. Add apricot jam, orange juice, and Dijon mustard to pan. Stir briefly. Pour over pork and serve.

EACH SERVING ABOUT: *358 calories, 30 g protein, 17 g carbohydrate, 19 g total fat (4 g saturated fat), 322 mg sodium, 16 mg calcium, 0 g fiber, 30 mg omega-3*

SIDES, SOUPS, SAUCES, AND SWEETS

GOOD FOR: *Heart, brain, strength, hair, nails, and teeth*

AMBROSIA PARFAITS

MAKES 4 dessert servings
PREP TIME 10 minutes

1 cup nonfat plain Greek yogurt
1 teaspoon orange zest
1½ cups pineapple chunks
2 seedless clementine oranges, peeled, separated into segments
1½ cups strawberries, halved
2 kiwis, peeled, halved lengthwise, cut into slices
¼ cup dried unsweetened coconut chips or shavings
Fresh mint leaves for garnish (optional)

1 In a medium bowl, whisk yogurt with orange zest. Set aside.
2 In a large bowl, combine pineapple, clementine segments, strawberries, kiwi, and coconut. Gently toss.
3 Spoon half of fruit mixture into dessert glasses. Cover with a large dollop of yogurt. Top with remaining fruit mixture. Garnish with mint leaves if desired.

EACH SERVING ABOUT: *157 calories, 7 g protein, 25 g carbohydrate, 4 g total fat (3 g saturated fat), 24 mg sodium, 106 mg calcium, 5 g fiber, 50 mg omega-3*

CANTALOUPE CUCUMBER SALAD

GOOD FOR: *Heart, skin*

MAKES 4 side-dish servings

PREP TIME 5 minutes

2 tablespoons lime juice
½ teaspoon kosher salt
¼ teaspoon ground black pepper
1½ cups diced cucumber
1 cantaloupe, coarsely chopped
1 scallion, sliced
2 tablespoons chopped cilantro

1 In a large bowl, whisk together lime juice, salt, and pepper.
2 Add cucumber, cantaloupe, scallion, and cilantro. Toss to coat.

EACH SERVING ABOUT: *60 calories, 1 g protein, 14 g carbohydrate, 0 g total fat (0 g saturated fat), 262 mg sodium, 32 mg calcium, 2 g fiber, 0 mg omega-3*

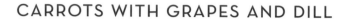

GF **V**

GOOD FOR: *Heart, cancer prevention, brain, and skin*

CARROTS WITH GRAPES AND DILL

MAKES 4 side-dish servings
PREP TIME 10 minutes
COOK TIME 10 minutes

1 pound carrots, peeled and cut into 1½-inch chunks
2 tablespoons olive oil
½ cup halved red seedless grapes
Large pinch kosher salt
1 tablespoon snipped fresh dill

1 Cook carrots uncovered in boiling water 8–10 minutes until crisp-tender. Drain.

2 In a medium saucepan, heat olive oil. Add carrots and stir until well coated. Stir in grapes and salt. Cook 2 minutes, or until hot. Sprinkle with dill.

EACH SERVING ABOUT: *117 calories, 2 g protein, 14 g carbohydrate, 7 g fat (1 g saturated fat), 148 mg sodium, 31 mg calcium, 3 g fiber, 0 mg omega-3*

CUMIN-SPICED PUMPKIN SOUP

LC **V**

GOOD FOR: *Heart, blood sugar, cancer prevention, and skin*

MAKES 4 1-cup servings
PREP TIME 5 minutes
COOK TIME 30 minutes

1 tablespoon unsalted butter
1 shallot, finely chopped
½ teaspoon cumin
15-ounce can pure pumpkin
2 cups reduced-sodium vegetable broth
½ cup water
¼ teaspoon kosher salt

1 In 4-quart saucepot, melt butter on medium-high. Add shallot, cook 30 seconds, stirring.
2 Add cumin, and cook 1 minute, stirring frequently. Add pumpkin, broth, and water.
3 Cover and heat to boiling on high. Stir in salt. Remove from heat.

EACH SERVING ABOUT: *76 calories, 2 g protein, 11 g carbohydrate, 3 g total fat (2 g saturated fat), 196 mg sodium, 31 mg calcium, 5 g fiber, 10 mg omega-3*

FROZEN FRUIT YOGURT

GOOD FOR: *Heart, blood sugar, cancer prevention, and brain*

MAKES 8 dessert servings
PREP TIME 10 minutes

2 ¾ cups frozen strawberries, cherries, or peaches
2 ½ cups frozen raspberries
1 cup nonfat plain Greek yogurt
2 tablespoons sugar
1 tablespoon fresh lemon juice
⅛ teaspoon almond extract

1   In a food processor with knife blade attached, blend frozen fruit until fruit resembles finely shaved ice, stopping processor occasionally to scrape down sides.

2   Add yogurt, sugar, lemon juice, and almond extract, and process just until mixture is smooth and creamy, scraping down sides occasionally. Serve immediately. Or, spoon into freezer-safe containers and freeze to serve later; let stand at room temperature 10 minutes to soften slightly before serving.

EACH SERVING ABOUT: *60 calories, 3 g protein, 13 g carbohydrate, 0 g total fat (0 g saturated fat), 10 mg sodium, 43 mg calcium, 3 g fiber, 0 mg omega-3*

ROASTED PEARS

GF **V**

GOOD FOR: *Heart, cancer prevention*

MAKES 4 dessert servings
PREP TIME 5 minutes
COOK TIME 30 minutes

4 pears, quartered and cored
2 tablespoons olive oil
4 teaspoons brown sugar
½ teaspoon cinnamon

1 Preheat oven to 400°F.
2 Brush pears with olive oil. Place on a baking sheet. Sprinkle with brown sugar and cinnamon.
3 Roast for 25 to 30 minutes, or until tender when pierced with a knife.

EACH SERVING ABOUT: *177 calories, 1 g protein, 31 g carbohydrate, 7 g fat (1 g saturated fat), 2 mg sodium, 19 mg calcium, 6 g fiber, 0 mg omega-3*

GOOD FOR: *Heart, blood sugar, cancer prevention, and skin*

SUMMER TOMATO SAUCE

MAKES 12 ½-cup servings
PREP TIME 20 minutes
COOK TIME 50 minutes

4 pounds fresh tomatoes
¼ cup olive oil
1 large yellow onion, finely chopped
4 cloves garlic, thinly sliced
1 teaspoon kosher salt
¼ teaspoon ground black pepper
1 cup basil leaves

1 Bring a large pot of water to a boil.
2 Meanwhile, fill a large bowl with water and ice. Using a paring knife, core each tomato and score a small X in bottom.
3 Working in batches, use a slotted spoon to carefully add tomatoes to boiling water. Let boil until skins begin to split, 15–30 seconds. Immediately transfer tomatoes to ice water.
4 Peel tomatoes and discard skins. Place a cutting board in a rimmed baking sheet. Cut tomatoes in half, squeeze out and discard seeds, then coarsely chop remaining tomato.
5 Heat oil in a large saucepan over medium heat. Add onion and cook, covered, stirring occasionally, until very tender, 10–12 minutes.
6 Add garlic and cook, stirring until soft, 1–2 minutes. Add tomatoes and their juices, salt, and pepper, and simmer, stirring occasionally, until tomatoes break down and sauce thickens, 35–40 minutes. Stir in basil. Serve immediately or freeze for up to 6 months.

EACH SERVING ABOUT: *83 calories, 1 g protein, 9 g carbohydrate, 5 g total fat (1 g saturated fat), 166 mg sodium, 32 mg calcium, 1 g fiber, 10 mg omega-3*

WATERMELON GRANITA

GOOD FOR: *Heart, cancer prevention, and skin*

MAKES 4 dessert servings
PREP TIME 5 minutes
WAITING TIME 2½ hours

3 cups cubed seedless watermelon
2 tablespoons sugar
2 tablespoons fresh lime juice

1   Purée watermelon in a food processor. Add sugar and lime juice. Pulse until sugar is dissolved.
2   Pour into a 9×13-inch baking pan. Freeze 2½ hours, stirring each hour, mixing ice crystals into middle of pan.
3   Remove granita from freezer. Let stand for 10 minutes at room temperature. Scrape into chilled glasses and serve at once.

EACH SERVING ABOUT: *60 calories, 1 g protein, 16 g carbohydrate, 0 g total fat (0 g saturated fat), 1 mg sodium, 9 mg calcium, 0 g fiber, 0 mg omega-3*

HEALTHY PUMPKIN BREAD

GOOD FOR: *Cancer prevention, brain, and skin*

MAKES 14 servings
PREP TIME 20 minutes
COOK TIME 1 hour 10 minutes

Nonstick cooking spray
1 cup plus 1 tablespoon all-purpose flour, divided use
1 cup brown sugar
2 egg whites
1 cup puréed pumpkin
¼ cup canola oil
⅓ cup plain nonfat yogurt
1 teaspoon vanilla extract
¾ cup whole-wheat flour
1½ teaspoon baking powder
1 teaspoon cinnamon
½ teaspoon ground nutmeg
½ teaspoon baking soda
½ teaspoon salt

1 Preheat oven to 350°F. Spray an 8½" by 4½" metal loaf pan with nonstick cooking spray and dust with 1 tablespoon all-purpose flour.

2 In large bowl, with wire whisk, combine brown sugar and egg whites. Add pumpkin, oil, yogurt, and vanilla extract; stir to combine.

3 In medium bowl, combine remaining all-purpose flour, whole-wheat flour, baking powder, cinnamon, nutmeg, baking soda, and salt. Add flour mixture to pumpkin mixture; stir until just combined. Do not overmix.

4 Pour batter into prepared pan. Bake 45 to 50 minutes or until toothpick inserted in center of loaf comes out clean. Cool in pan 10 minutes. Invert pumpkin bread onto wire rack; cool completely.

EACH SERVING ABOUT: *143 calories, 3 g protein, 24 g carbohydrate, 4 g total fat (0 g saturated fat), 144 mg sodium, 87 mg calcium, 2 g fiber, 370 mg omega-3*

SNACKS

GOOD FOR: *Heart, blood sugar, strength, hair, nails, and teeth*

CHEESY CORN TORTILLAS

MAKES 1 serving

Top one **6-inch corn tortilla** with **¼ cup shredded part-skim mozzarella cheese**. Heat in microwave for 30–60 seconds or until cheese melts.

EACH SERVING ABOUT: *135 calories, 9 g protein, 12 g carbohydrate, 5 g total fat (2 g saturated fat), 203 mg sodium, 200 mg calcium, 1 g fiber, 0 mg omega-3*

V

GOOD FOR: *Heart, blood sugar, cancer prevention, brain, strength, skin, hair, nails, and teeth*

CHIA PUDDING

MAKES 1 serving

In a small bowl, combine **2 tablespoons chia seeds** with **2/3 cup unsweetened vanilla almond milk** and **1 tablespoon chopped dried apricots**. Stir well. Cover and chill overnight in refrigerator.

EACH SERVING ABOUT: *150 calories, 4 g protein, 16 g carbohydrate, 8 g total fat (1 g saturated fat), 129 mg sodium, 273 mg calcium, 8 g fiber, 3,740 mg omega-3*

GOOD FOR: *Heart, blood sugar, cancer prevention, brain, skin*

CHOCOLATE CHILI POPCORN

MAKES 1 serving

In a large zip-top bag, combine **4 cups air-popped or lowfat microwave popcorn** with **1 teaspoon unsweetened cocoa powder** and **1 large pinch chili powder**. Shake well to coat.

EACH SERVING ABOUT: *141 calories, 4 g protein, 25 g carbohydrate, 3 g total fat (0 g saturated fat), 283 mg sodium, 4 mg calcium, 5 g fiber, 80 mg omega-3*

GOOD-FOR-YOU HOT CHOCOLATE

MAKES 1 serving

GOOD FOR: *Heart, strength, skin, hair, nails, and teeth*

Pour **8 ounces 1% milk** into a large mug. Whisk in **2 teaspoons unsweetened cocoa powder** and **2 teaspoons sugar**. Stir well. Microwave for 1 minute or until heated through.

EACH SERVING ABOUT: *149 calories, 10 g protein, 23 g carbohydrate, 3 g total fat (2 g saturated fat), 130 mg sodium, 300 mg calcium, 1 g fiber, 0 mg omega-3*

PB & BANANA "SANDWICH"

MAKES 1 serving

GOOD FOR: *Heart, cancer prevention, brain, skin*

Slice **½ medium banana** crosswise. Spread bottom half with **1 tablespoon peanut butter**. Sprinkle with **a dash of cinnamon sugar**. Top with remaining banana half.

EACH SERVING ABOUT: *148 calories, 4 g protein, 18 g carbohydrate, 8 g total fat (2 g saturated fat), 77 mg sodium, 13 mg calcium, 3 g fiber, 20 mg omega 3*

PUMPKIN SMOOTHIE

MAKES 1 serving

GOOD FOR: *Heart, cancer prevention, skin, hair, nails, and teeth*

In a blender, combine **¾ cup of kefir**, **½ cup frozen pineapple chunks**, **½ cup canned pumpkin purée**, and **1 pinch ground ginger** for 1½–2 minutes or until smooth.

EACH SERVING ABOUT: *145 calories, 9 g protein, 24 g carbohydrates, 2 g total fat (1 g saturated fat), 98 mg sodium, 252 mg calcium, 3 g fiber, 20 mg omega-3.*

GOOD FOR: *Heart, blood sugar, cancer prevention, strength, skin*

SPICY TRAIL MIX

MAKES 1 serving

In a sandwich-size zip-top bag, combine **1 tablespoon pumpkin seeds**, **2 tablespoons roasted soybeans**, **1 tablespoon dried tart cherries**, and **a dash each of cayenne pepper and cinnamon**. Seal bag and shake well to combine.

EACH SERVING ABOUT: *143 calories, 7 g protein, 12 g carbohydrate, 8 g total fat (1 g saturated fat), 2 mg sodium, 22 mg calcium, 3 g fiber, 170 mg omega-3*

GOOD FOR: *Heart, cancer prevention, brain, strength, skin, hair, nails, and teeth*

STRAWBERRY SMOOTHIE

MAKES 1 serving

In a blender, combine **½ cup nonfat plain Greek yogurt**, **1 cup frozen strawberries**, **¼ cup orange juice**, and **½ teaspoon honey** for 1½–2 minutes or until smooth.

EACH SERVING ABOUT: *144 calories, 12 g protein, 27 g carbohydrate, 0 g total fat (0 g saturated fat), 43 mg sodium, 101 mg calcium, 3 g fiber, 10 mg omega-3*

MEAL PLANS

Master meal plan

	BREAKFAST	LUNCH	DINNER
DAY 1	Breakfast Burrito*	Kale Salad with Chicken and Cheddar*	Lemon Pasta with Salmon and Asparagus*
DAY 2	Cantaloupe Breakfast Bowl*	Curried Chickpea Pita*	Cashew-Chicken Stir-Fry* 2 clementines
DAY 3	Tropical Greek Yogurt Breakfast Parfait*	Sardine, Cucumber, and Endive Sandwich*	Orange-Soy Tofu Stir-Fry* 1/3 cup quinoa prepared according to package directions
DAY 4	Better-for-You Blueberry Waffles*	Brown Rice Edamame Salad*	Roast Pork Tenderloin with Blackberry Sauce* 1/4 cup whole-wheat couscous prepared according to package directions 1/2 cup broccoli florets sautéed in 1 teaspoon olive oil
DAY 5	Maple Almond Oatmeal*	Couscous with Chickpeas*	Greek-Style Tilapia* 3/4 cup peas tossed with 1 teaspoon olive oil Watermelon Granita*
DAY 6	Spinach-Feta Omelet* 1 medium orange	Salmon Pesto Sandwich* 1/4 cup rinsed and drained no-salt-added canned chickpeas with 1 cup sliced cherry tomatoes and 1 teaspoon balsamic vinegar	Grilled Chicken Salad with Avocado and Grapefruit* 1 small (1 ounce) whole-wheat dinner roll
DAY 7	Pomegranate-Apricot Breakfast Crostini*	Quinoa Cannellini Salad*	Spice-Roasted Chicken, Red Onions, Carrots, and Parsnips* 1 cup mixed berries

*Recipe included in chapter 9

Chia Pudding*

Unlimited vegetables dipped in ¾ cup nonfat plain yogurt mixed with a large pinch curry powder

Cheesy Corn Tortillas*

3 2-inch cinnamon graham squares, each topped with 2 tablespoons part-skim ricotta and drizzled with ¼ teaspoon honey

Good-for-You Hot Chocolate*

1 hardboiled egg sprinkled with chili powder + 8 small whole-grain crackers

Pumpkin Smoothie*

2 tablespoons walnuts mixed with 2 tablespoons dried tart cherries

PB & Banana "Sandwich"*

6 ounces nonfat plain Greek yogurt with ½ cup blueberries

12-ounce nonfat latte (6 ounces nonfat milk warmed in the microwave + 6 ounces hot brewed coffee) + ¾ cup grapes

Spicy Trail Mix*

Strawberry Smoothie*

1 apple and 2 1-inch Brie cubes

In the pages of this book, you've read about a lot of age-defying Super Nutrients. This 1-week comprehensive meal plan is packed with recipes featuring Power Foods that provide all the nutrients you need to look and feel healthier, stronger, and more energetic.

Gluten-free meal plan

	BREAKFAST	LUNCH	DINNER
DAY 1	Apricot Ricotta Breakfast Sundae*	Baked Potato "Burrito Bowl"*	Greek-Style Tilapia* (substitute 1 cup quinoa for whole-wheat couscous) ½ cup grapes with 2 1-inch cubes Brie cheese
DAY 2	Huevos Rancheros*	Quinoa Cannellini Salad	Chicken Vegetable Skewers* Roasted Pears*
DAY 3	Orange and Apricot Quinoa*	Apple Spinach Salad*	Cauliflower Curry Stew*
DAY 4	Spinach-Feta Omelet* 1 medium orange	Brown Rice–Stuffed Pepper (swap in brown rice for barley in Barley-Stuffed Pepper*) 1 medium apple	Garlic Shrimp and Swiss Chard on Polenta*
DAY 5	Tropical Greek Yogurt Breakfast Parfait*	Quinoa with Chickpeas (swap in quinoa for couscous in Couscous with Chickpeas*)	Spice-Roasted Chicken, Red Onions, Carrots, and Parsnips* 1 cup mixed berries
DAY 6	Peach Blueberry Smoothie*	Kale Salad with Chicken and Cheddar* (if you can't find gluten-free Worcestershire sauce, simply omit it)	Mexican Burrito Bowl*
DAY 7	Cantaloupe Breakfast Bowl*	Tuna Fennel Wrap* (swap in two 6-inch corn tortillas for the whole-wheat tortilla)	Slow Cooker African Sweet Potato–Peanut Stew*

*Recipe included in chapter 9

Cheesy Corn Tortillas*
Spicy Trail Mix*

Chocolate Chili Popcorn*
12-ounce nonfat latte (6 ounces nonfat milk warmed in the microwave + 6 ounces hot brewed coffee) + 3/4 cup grapes

Spicy Trail Mix*
Good-for-You Hot Chocolate*

45 pistachio nuts
Pumpkin Smoothie*

2 tablespoons walnuts mixed with 2 tablespoons dried tart cherries
6 ounces nonfat plain Greek yogurt with 1/2 cup blueberries

PB & Banana "Sandwich"*
Unlimited vegetables dipped in 3/4 cup nonfat plain yogurt mixed with a large pinch curry powder

Strawberry Smoothie*
17 cashew nuts

Whether you have celiac disease or you're just trying to avoid gluten, this meal plan will ensure you're consuming all of the Super Nutrients and Power Foods you need for optimal health and longevity.

➤ GOOD TO KNOW! *If you're avoiding gluten, be sure to read the ingredient list on all packaged foods such as chicken broth or deli turkey. While these are often gluten-free, ingredients can vary from brand to brand.*

Low-carb meal plan

	BREAKFAST	LUNCH	DINNER
DAY 1	Apricot Ricotta Breakfast Sundae*	BBQ Turkey Burger*	Steak and Onion Tacos with Fresh Tomato Salsa* Serve topped with ⅓ avocado, diced
DAY 2	Spinach-Feta Omelet* 1 medium orange	Grilled Shrimp Caesar* 40 pistachio nuts	Roast Pork Tenderloin with Blackberry Sauce* (enjoy two servings!)
DAY 3	Avocado Swiss Breakfast Sandwich*	Kale Salad with Chicken and Cheddar*	Sesame Salmon with Bok Choy* 1 cup edamame in their pods
DAY 4	Cantaloupe Breakfast Bowl* (omit blueberries and add in 2 tablespoons almonds)	Veggie Burger Parmesan* 1 cup arugula drizzled with 2 teaspoons each olive oil and red wine vinegar	Spice-Roasted Chicken, Red Onions, Carrots, and Parsnips* 1 cup of arugula with 2 teaspoons each olive oil and red wine vinegar
DAY 5	Crunchy Sunflower Butter Sandwich* (use only ½ apple and increase sunflower butter to 1½ tablespoons)	Asian Chicken Tacos*	Orange-Soy Tofu Stir-Fry* Microwave ½ ounce dark chocolate for 30 seconds to 1 minute; drizzle over 12 pecan halves
DAY 6	Huevos Rancheros*	Salmon Pesto Sandwich* topped with ¼ sliced avocado	Turkey Cutlets Piccata* ¾ cup of cooked peas tossed in 2 teaspoons olive oil 1 cup sliced strawberries
DAY 7	Tropical Greek Yogurt Breakfast Parfait*	Tuna Cheddar Melt* ¾ cup cubed cantaloupe	Spiced Pork Tenderloins with Mango Salsa* (enjoy two servings!) 1 cup steamed asparagus drizzled with 1 teaspoon olive oil

*Recipe included in chapter 9

SNACKS
Spicy Trail Mix* 2 pieces lowfat string cheese
1 cup sliced fennel dipped in ¼ cup hummus 6 ounces nonfat plain Greek yogurt mixed with 1 pinch cinnamon and topped with ½ cup strawberries
15 pecan halves 1 hardboiled egg sprinkled with curry powder + 8 small whole-grain crackers
1 cup 1% cottage cheese mixed with chopped fresh herbs like parsley or tarragon ¾ cup edamame
Unlimited broccoli and cauliflower florets dipped in 1 tablespoon ranch dressing 1 apple + 2 1-inch Brie cubes
6 large olives, 1 1-inch cube feta cheese, and 1 cup sliced red and yellow peppers 23 almonds
1 large celery stalk filled with 1½ tablespoons nut butter Cheesy Corn Tortillas*

Looking to eat fewer carbs to help control your blood sugar or to slim down? This plan is for you. Each meal and snack provides no more than 35 and 15 grams of carbohydrates, respectively.

Vegetarian meal plan

	BREAKFAST	LUNCH	DINNER
DAY 1	Gooey Strawberry French Toast*	Broccoli and Tomato Pizza*	Mexican Burrito Bowl*
DAY 2	Crunchy Sunflower Butter Sandwich*	Mediterranean Pasta Salad*	Slow Cooker Italian Lentil and Vegetable Stew* Melt 1 tablespoon dark chocolate chips in the microwave for 30 seconds and drizzle over 1/2 cup sliced strawberries.
DAY 3	Creamy Orange Banana Waffle*	Black Bean Burger Salad*	Cauliflower Mac 'n' Cheese*
DAY 4	Breakfast Burrito*	Veggie Burger Parmesan* 1 cup arugula drizzled with 2 teaspoons each olive oil and balsamic vinaigrette	Orange-Soy Tofu Stir-Fry* 1/3 cup quinoa prepared according to package directions
DAY 5	Avocado Swiss Breakfast Sandwich*	Brown Rice Edamame Salad*	Pasta with Asparagus, Cannellini, and Parmesan*
DAY 6	Huevos Rancheros*	Barley-Stuffed Pepper* 1 medium pear	Spaghetti with Beets, Greens, and Ricotta*
DAY 7	Sunrise Smoothie*	Couscous with Chickpeas*	Slow Cooker Butternut Squash Barley Risotto* 1 cup arugula with 1/2 cup cannellini beans and 1 tablespoon balsamic vinaigrette

*Recipe included in chapter 9

SNACKS
3 2-inch cinnamon graham squares, each topped with 2 tablespoons part-skim ricotta and drizzled with ¼ teaspoon honey 1 nut-based snack bar
Spicy Trail Mix* Unlimited vegetables dipped in ¾ cup nonfat plain yogurt mixed with a large pinch curry powder
12-ounce nonfat green tea latte (6 ounces soy milk warmed in the microwave + 6 ounces hot green tea + 1 tsp honey) Chia Pudding*
1 container lowfat vanilla yogurt with ¼ cup pomegranate seeds 1 apple with 1 tablespoon nut butter
¾ cup edamame Pumpkin Smoothie*
1 ounce dark chocolate 12-ounce nonfat latte + 2 kiwi
1 hardboiled egg sprinkled with curry powder + 8 small whole-grain crackers 1 sliced bell pepper dipped in 1 tablespoon tahini

If you're a vegetarian, you may need to pay extra attention to certain nutrients, such as iron, zinc, vitamin B12, and protein. This plant-based plan shows you how to get these—along with all the other Super Nutrients you need to beat aging.

ANTI-AGING EXPERT SOURCES

Elliott Antman, M.D. is a Senior Physician, Brigham and Women's Hospital and Associate Dean for Clinical and Translational Research, Harvard Medical School.

Constance Brown-Riggs, MSEd, R.D., C.D.E., C.D.N. is the author of *The African American Guide to Living Well With Diabetes* and a board member of the American Association of Diabetes Educators.

Karen Collins, M.S., R.D.N., C.D.N., F.A.N.D. is a nationally syndicated nutrition news columnist, speaker, consultant and a nutrition advisor for the American Institute for Cancer Research.

Alessio Fasano, M.D. is the Director of the Center for Celiac Research at Massachusetts General Hospital.

Mario Ferruzzi, Ph.D. is a Professor of Food Science and Nutrition at Purdue University.

Balz Frei, Ph.D. is the director emeritus of the Linus Pauling Institute and a distinguished professor emeritus at Oregon State University.

Francesca Fusco, M.D. is a dermatologist specializing in hair and scalp health with Wexler Dermatology in New York City and an assistant clinical professor of dermatology at Mount Sinai Medical Center.

Jeannette Graf, M.D. is an Assistant Clinical Professor of Dermatology at Mount Sinai Medical Center in New York City and the author of *Stop Aging, Start Living: The Revolutionary 2-Week pH Diet That Erases Wrinkles, Beautifies Skin, and Makes You Feel Fantastic.*

Kimberly Harms, D.D.S. is a consumer advisor for the American Dental Association.

Michael Holick, Ph.D., M.D. is a Professor of Medicine, Physiology and Biophysics at Boston University School of Medicine and author of *The Vitamin D Solution: A 3-Step Strategy to Cure Our Most Common Health Problems.*

Rachel Johnson, Ph.D., M.P.H., R.D. is the Robert L. Bickford Jr. Green and Gold Professor of Nutrition at the University of Vermont and past chair of the American Heart Association's Nutrition Committee.

David Katz, M.D. is the Founding Director Yale-Griffin Prevention Research Center and author of *Disease Proof: The Remarkable Truth About What Keeps Us Well*.

David Kingsley, Ph.D. is a New York City trichologist who treats hair and scalp conditions, as well as the creator of British Science Formulations products for thinning hair.

Penny Kris-Etherton, Ph.D., R.D. is a Distinguished Professor of Nutrition at Penn State University and a fellow of both the American Heart Association and the American Lipid Association.

Meghan O'Brien, M.D. is a Clinical Instructor of Dermatology at Weill Cornell Medical Center in New York City and dermatologist with Tribeca Park Dermatology.

Douglas Paddon-Jones, Ph.D. is a professor in the Department of Nutrition and Metabolism at the University of Texas Medical Branch.

Melissa Peck Piliang, M.D. is the Associate Program Director of Dermatology Residency with the Cleveland Clinic Foundation.

Nicole E. Rogers M.D., F.A.A.D is a hair transplant surgeon and Assistant Clinical Professor of Dermatology at Tulane University.

Joan Salge Blake, M.S., R.D., L.D.N. is a Clinical Associate Professor at Boston University's Sargent College of Health and Rehabilitation.

Barbara Shukitt Hale, Ph.D. is a Research Psychologist with the Jean Mayer USDA Human Nutrition Research Center on Aging at Tufts University.

Victoria Stevens, Ph.D. is the Strategic Director, Laboratory Services for the American Cancer Society.

Katherine L. Tucker, Ph.D. is a Professor of Nutritional Epidemiology at the University of Massachusetts at Lowell.

INDEX